30 Day Whole Foods Cookbook

90 Whole Recipes for YOUR Healthy Life

(breakfast, lunch, dinner)

Stella Parker

Table of Contents

Introduction

The concept of the Whole Foods diet dates back to early 2009 when medicinal practitioners Melissa Hartwig and Dallas Hartwig first introduced the program to the world.

The core aim of a Whole Foods diet is to completely reset the nutritional values of the body within a span of 30 days and put an end to unhealthy eating habits while helping to restore and reinvigorate the body's metabolic, digestive and diseases preventive functionalities.

And how does it do that?

Well, there's no magical formula behind all of it! Just like any other diet out there, Whole Foods also requires you to completely give up specific food groups (such as junk foods, sugary foods, and dairy products) which are believed to negatively impact the well- being of your body if taken in large quantities.

Since the diet is essentially eliminating these kind of produces for 30 days, the diet is also sometimes referred to as Elimination Diet.

To quote the founders and designers of the Whole Foods program, "By eliminating all of the inflammatory, psychology unhealthy, gut-disrupting and hormone unbalancing foods groups for 30 days, the Whole Foods diet will literally 'Change Your Life' forever!"

You might be wondering, though, that this diet essentially sounds like a Paleo or Atkins Diet! The reason for that is because Whole Foods Is actually based on the framework of a Paleo diet.

However,

Do I have your attention now? Excellent!

Allow me to educate you further on the topic of Whole Foods now before you jump in on the recipes and start to "Change Your Life."

The Benefits of Whole Foods

Now obviously you would not want to go headfirst into a completely new diet without knowing a little bit about the possible outcomes of the diet right?

So, instead of putting this section at the end of the chapter like many other diet books, I am going to share the benefits of the diet upfront, which should inspire you further to mentally prepare yourself for the journey ahead.

- If sugar is eliminated from your system, you will be able to get more sound and relaxing sleep.
- You'll be able to get a boost of consistent energy all throughout the day.
- You won't be facing any digestive problems such as stomach bloating, farts or tummy rumblings.
- You will be at peace and your anxiety levels will significantly lower down.
- The condition of your skin will vastly improve since you are going for more vegetables and protein while eliminating sugar altogether.
- Your hair will be healthier and shinier.
- Workout sessions will be more effective.
- Not to mention, aside from making you healthy! The Whole Foods diet will actually help you to trim down that pesky

body fat and give you a fine body image and attractive physique.

Hyped up enough?

At that's just the tip of the Ice Berg! If you are dedicated enough to embark on the journey of Whole Foods, then you might be surprised by how much better your life becomes.

That being said, let us now have a look at a general list of foods that are allowed on this diet.

Foods that are allowed for Whole Foods

- Almond flour
- Almond milk
- Arrowroot Powder
- Bacon
- Bean Sprouts
- Cacao
- Canola Oil
- Olive Oil
- Carob
- Chia
- Citric Acid
- Coconut Flour
- Coconut Water
- Coffee
- Dates
- Flax Seed
- Fruit Juice
- Guar Gum
- Green Beans
- Hemp Seeds
- Larabars
- Mayonnaise (Homemade)
- Mustard
- Nutritional Yeast
- Potatoes (Added in August 2014)
- Salt
- Sunflower Oil
- Snow Peas

- Tahini
- Water Kefir

And the foods that are completely restricted!

Foods that not are allowed for Whole Foods

- Amino Acids
- Buckwheat
- Carob
- Deep Fried Chips
- Dark Chocolate
- Chewing Gum
- Hummus
- Paleo Bread
- Paleo Ice Cream
- Pancakes
- Any kind of Protein Shakes
- Quinoa
- Stevia Leaf
- Vanilla Extract

No side effects of Whole Foods?

If you have experimented a number of different diets before joining the Whole Foods tribe, then you have most probably seen that there are at least "some" side effects accompanying them.

You might be wondering if the Whole Foods also has some hidden side effects as well.

The good news is that with the Whole Foods, you won't be facing any serious side effects. However, there have been reports of some temporary symptoms which are normal for newcomers.

Just so that you don't get alarmed if you fall prey to any of these! Here is a list of the most common symptoms which you might face while following a Whole Foods Diet, which is very normal and is nothing to be afraid of.

These symptoms usually show up within the first 14 days of the diet and soon goes away once the body habituates itself to the new diet.

- Minor headaches
- Feeling of lethargy
- Sleepiness
- General Crankiness
- Brain Fog
- Food Cravings

- Minor Breakouts
- Minor Bloating

With all of those out of the way, here are some tips which you should keep in mind in order to make your Whole Foods journey as pleasant as possible.

10 amazing tips for Whole Foods

- Make up your mind and only start if you are fully committed.
- Instead of thinking of the 30 days as a whole, plan out the first 2 weeks first. Then go for the next 2 weeks.
- Clear out your house off all foods that are unsuitable for Whole Foods.
- Plan your meals beforehand.
- Mix and match to create your very own food schedule that will keep you entertained throughout the month.
- Make sure to keep one day aside to create your meal plan for the rest of the week.
- Keep your food related socializing events at a minimum.
- The Whole Foods community is full of inspiration stories and figures. If you ever start feeling left out, just browse the web, and you will get a plethora of support materials.
- Try to keep yourself distracted from food cravings.
- And most importantly, never give up!

Chapter 1: 30 Breakfast Ideas

Breakfast Idea #1 - The Perfect Whole Foods Baked Egg

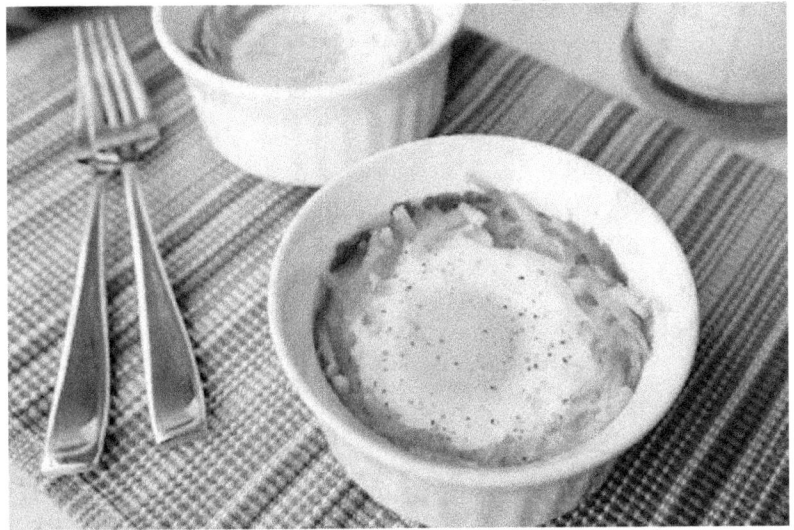

Prep Time: 10 minutes

Cooking Time: 30 minutes

Serving: 4

Ingredients:

- 1 cup water
- 1 cup marinara sauce
- 4 eggs

Directions:

1. Pre-heat your oven to a temperature of 350 degrees Fahrenheit
2. Take a kettle and pour water in it
3. Heat it up until it begins to steam

4. Remove the heat and pour 1 cup of the steaming water into the bottom of a nice casserole dish
5. Take 2-3 ramekins(depending on your serving)
6. Pour ¼ cup of marinara sauce into each of the ramekins
7. Crack 1 egg in each of the ramekins
8. Arrange the ramekin in your casserole dish
9. Fill up the dish with just enough water to reach the midpoint of each of the ramekin
10. Bake in your pre-heated oven for 25 minutes until the yolks are nicely firm
11. Serve!

Nutrition:

- Calories: 126
- Fat: 6.7g
- Carbohydrates: 9g
- Protein: 7.4g

Breakfast Idea #2 - Roasted Beets With Sautéed Beet Greens

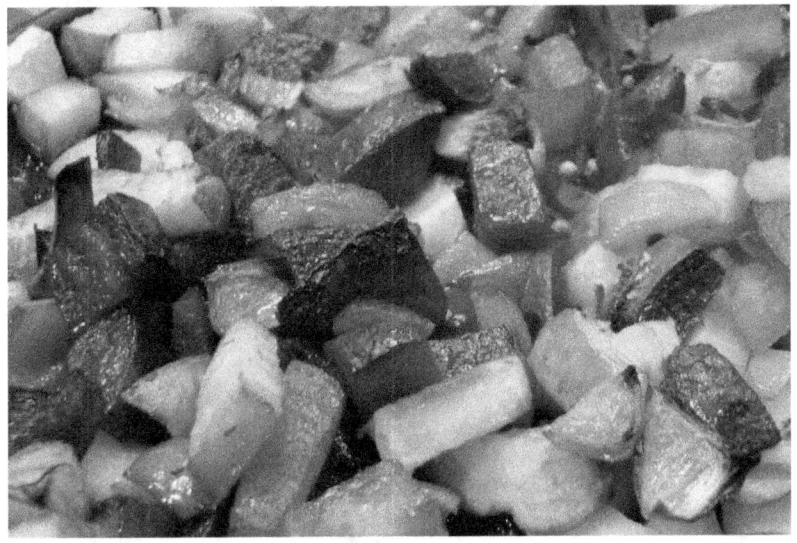

Prep Time: 10 minutes

Cooking Time: 30 minutes

Serving: 4

Ingredients:

- 1 bunch beets with greens
- ¼ cup divide olive oil
- 2 minced garlic cloves
- 2 tablespoon chopped onion
- Salt as needed
- Pepper as needed
- 1 tablespoon red wine vinegar

Directions:

1. Pre-heat your oven to a temperature of 350 degrees Fahrenheit
2. Wash up your beets thoroughly, making sure to keep the skin on
3. Remove the greens and rinse them up separately, making sure to remove any large stem
4. Keep them on the side
5. Place your beets in a small sized baking dish and toss them with 2 tablespoons of olive oil until finely coated
6. Cover it up and bake them for about 45-60 minutes in your oven
7. Once the beets are done, take a skillet over medium-low heat and pour 2 tablespoons of olive oil
8. Add garlic, onion and cook it for another minute
9. Tear up the beet greens into 2-3 inch pieces and add them to the skillet
10. Cook and keep stirring until the greens are soft and wilted
11. Season them with pepper and salt
12. Serve the green as they are
13. Serve the beets by seasoning them with some salt/pepper, butter or red-wine vinegar

Nutrition:

- Calories: 204
- Fat: 13g
- Carbohydrates: 18g
- Protein: 5.3g

Breakfast Idea #3 - Chicken Puttanesca In 30 Minutes!

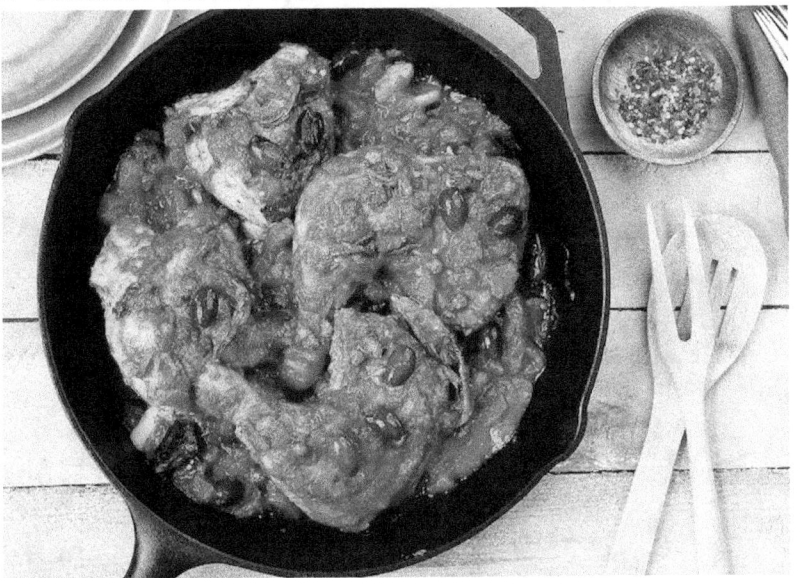

Prep Time: 15 minutes

Cooking Time: 20 minutes

Serving: 4

Ingredients:

- 4-5 pieces boneless chicken breast
- 1 tablespoon olive oil
- 1 cup halved and sliced onion
- 3 roughly chopped up garlic cloves
- 14 ounce crushed tomatoes
- 1 cup cherry tomatoes
- ½ a cup pitted kalamata olives
- ¼ cup chopped fresh basil
- Salt as needed
- Pepper as needed

Directions:

1. Take a large sized skillet and pour in the olive oil
2. Heat it up
3. Gently rinse your chicken and pat it dry using a kitchen towel
4. Add the chicken to the heated pan and brown it for 3-4 minutes on either side
5. Remove the chicken from the pan
6. Add the onions and Sauté for 1 minute
7. Add garlic and cook for another 1 minute
8. Add the basil and crushed tomatoes
9. Season the mix with some pepper and salt
10. Nestle the breast on top of your prepared sauce
11. Spread some olives and cherry tomatoes on top of the mix
12. Simmer for 20 minutes without the lid
13. Once thoroughly cooked, garnish with some basil
14. Serve!

Nutrition:

- Calories: 300
- Fat: 9.1g
- Carbohydrates: 19.9g
- Protein: 33g

Breakfast Idea #4 - Deliciously Roasted Okra

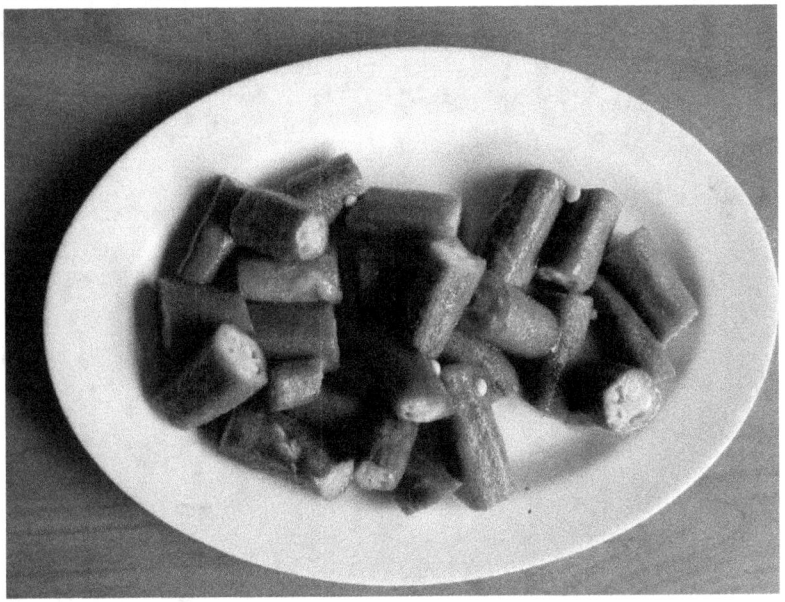

Prep Time: 5 minutes

Cooking Time: 15 minutes

Serving: 2

Ingredients:

- 18 fresh okra pods sliced up into 1/3 inch thick slices
- 1 tablespoon olive oil
- 2 teaspoon kosher salt
- 2 teaspoon black pepper

Directions:

1. Pre-heat your oven to a temperature of 425 degrees Fahrenheit

2. Arrange the okra slices in one layer on a nice cookie sheet lined with foil
3. Drizzle some olive oil over them
4. Sprinkle some pepper and salt
5. Bake in your pre-heated oven for about 10-15 minutes
6. Serve hot!

Nutrition:

- Calories: 65
- Fat: 4.6g
- Carbohydrates: 5.9g
- Protein: 1.6g

Breakfast Idea #5 – Whole Foods appreciated Cinnamon Coffee

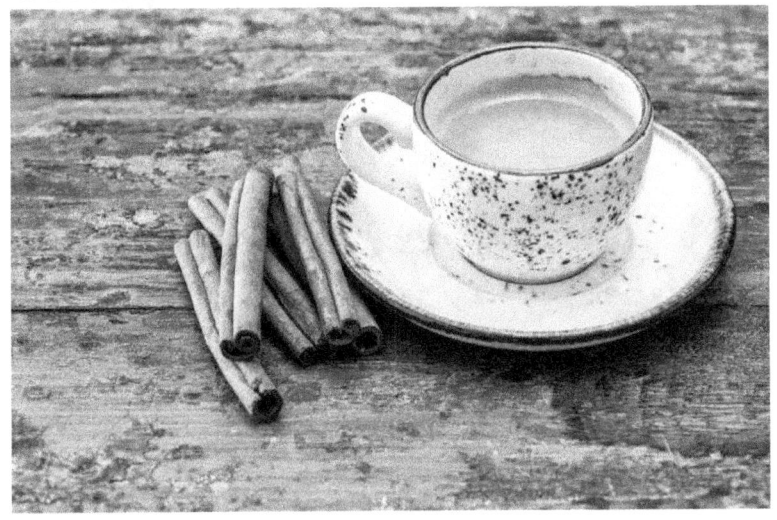

Prep Time: 5 minutes

Cooking Time: 10 minutes

Serving: 2

Ingredients:

- 2 tablespoon ground
- 1 teaspoon ground cinnamon
- 10 ounce hot water

Directions:

1. Take a small sized bowl and add cinnamon and coffee
2. Pour the hot water
3. Let it brew for 5 minutes
4. Strain into your favorite mug

5. Drink up!

Nutrition:

- Calories: 12
- Fat: 0g
- Carbohydrates: 3g
- Protein: 0.4g

Breakfast Idea #6 - Crispy And Juicy Macadamia Nutty Chicken

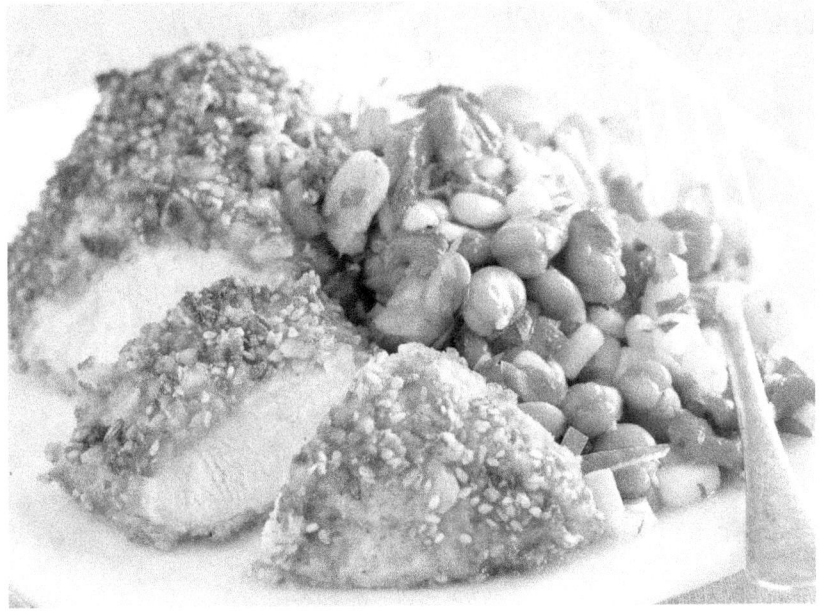

Prep Time: 10 minutes

Cooking Time: 30 minutes

Serving: 4

Ingredients:

- 3 pieces fine chicken breasts
- 2.3 ounce Macadamia Nuts
- 2 tablespoon homemade (Whole Foods) applicant mayonnaise

Directions:

1. Pre-heat your oven to a temperature of 400 degrees Fahrenheit

2. Gently wash your chicken breasts and pat them dry in a kitchen towel
3. Brush up the top side of your chicken breast with a light coat of mayo
4. Chop up the macadamia nuts and sprinkle them all over the chicken breasts
5. Bake for about 30 minutes in your pre-heated oven, making sure that the nuts are showing a brown texture
6. Serve with some extra mayo or Whole Foods compliant Dijon Mustard!

Nutrition:

- Calories: 1240
- Fat: 103g
- Carbohydrates: 45g
- Protein: 41g

Breakfast Idea #7 - The Perfect Tomatillo Salsa Verde

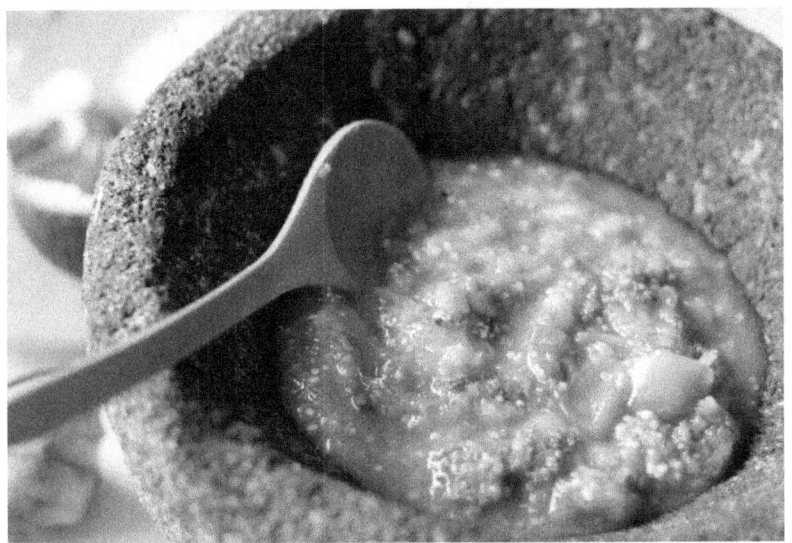

Prep Time: 10 minutes

Cooking Time: 15 minutes

Serving: 24

Ingredients:

- 1 cup water
- 1 cup marinara sauce
- 4 eggs

Directions:

1. Take a saucepan and add onions, tomatillos, chili pepper and garlic
2. Season with some oregano, cilantro, salt and cumin
3. Pour in the water

4. Bring the water to a boil over high temperature
5. Once boiling point is reached, lower down the heat to medium-low and simmer for 10-15 minutes until fully soft
6. Take a blender and pour the mix
7. Puree the mix until smooth
8. Serve with your favorite dipper!

Nutrition:

- Calories: 24
- Fat: 0.6g
- Carbohydrates: 4.6g
- Protein: 0.8g

Breakfast Idea #8 - Yours Truly, Carrot Soup!

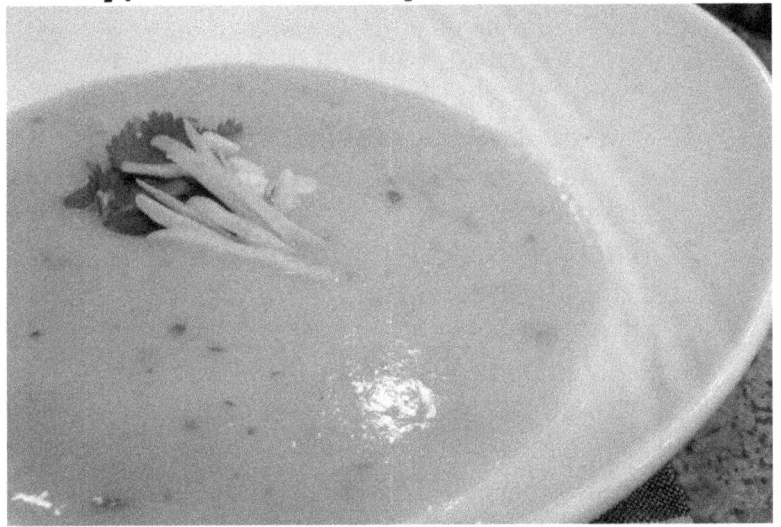

Prep Time: 15 minutes

Cooking Time: 25 minutes

Serving: 24

Ingredients:

- 2 tablespoon vegetable oil
- 1 chopped up onion
- 1 tablespoon curry powder
- 2 pound chopped up carrots
- 4 cups vegetable broth
- 2 cups water

Directions:

1. Take a large sized pot and place it over medium heat
2. Heat up the oil

3. Add onions and Sautee them until soft and translucent
4. Stir in your curry powder and add the chopped up carrots
5. Keep stirring the carrots until they are finely coated
6. Pour in the vegetable broth and simmer for another 20 minutes until the carrots are tender
7. Transfer the carrots alongside the broth to a blender and blend them until a smooth puree is formed
8. Pour it back into the pot
9. Add some water to get your preferred consistency
10. Serve hot!

Nutrition:

- Calories: 133
- Fat: 5.4g
- Carbohydrates: 20g
- Protein: 2.4g

Breakfast Idea #9 - Assorted Vegetable Roast To Start Your Day

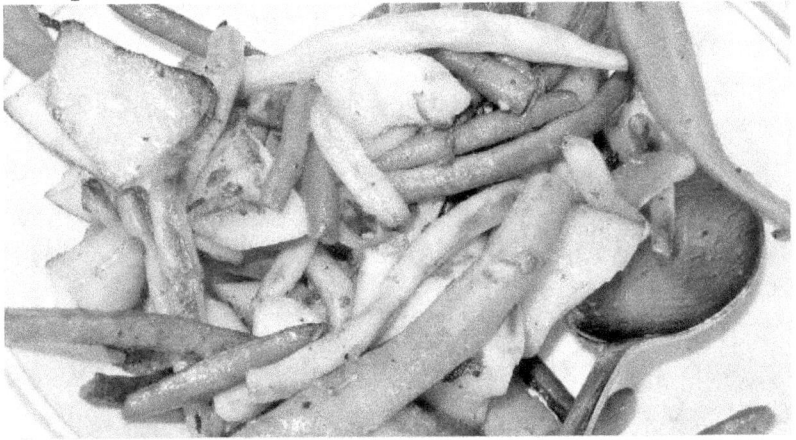

Prep Time: 15 minutes

Cooking Time: 40 minutes

Serving: 12

Ingredients:

- 1 small cubed of butternut squash
- 2 seeded and diced red bell peppers
- 1 peeled and cubed sweet potato
- 3 cubed Yukon Gold Potatoes
- 1 quartered red onion
- 1 tablespoon chopped fresh thyme
- 2 tablespoon chopped fresh rosemary
- ¼ cup of olive oil
- 2 tablespoon balsamic vinegar
- Salt as needed
- Ground black pepper as needed

Directions:

1. Pre-heat your oven to a temperature of 475 degrees Fahrenheit
2. Take a large sized bowl and add squash, sweet potato, red bell peppers and Yukon Gold Potatoes
3. Gently separate the red onion quarters into individual pieces and add them to the mix as well
4. Take a small bowl and stir the rosemary, thyme, vinegar, olive oil, pepper, and salt
5. Add the mix to the large bowl
6. Toss the vegetables finely until they are well coated
7. Tale a large sized roasting pan and spread the mix evenly
8. Roast for about 35-40 minutes in your pre-heated oven, making sure to keep stirring it for every 10 minutes
9. Serve hot!

Nutrition:

- Calories: 123
- Fat: 4.7g
- Carbohydrates: 20g
- Protein: 2g

Breakfast Idea #10 - Homemade Greek Dressing For Any Morning Salad

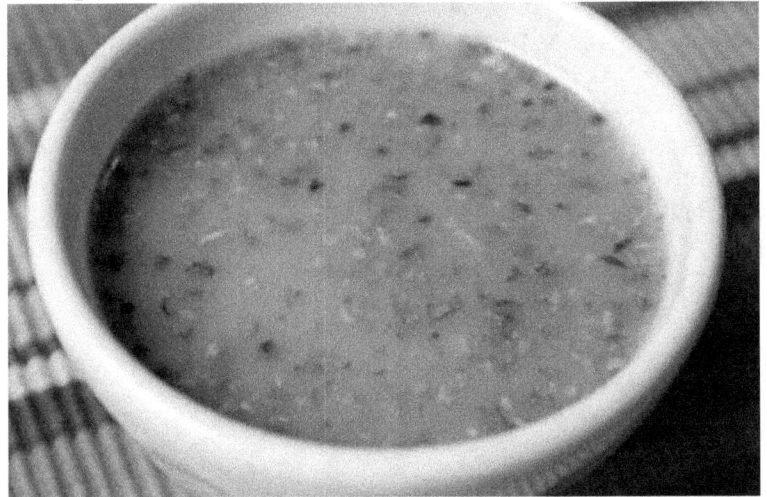

Prep Time: 10 minutes

Cooking Time: 10 minutes

Serving: 120

Ingredients:

- 1 and ½ quarts of olive oil
- 1/3 cup garlic powder
- 1/3 cup dried oregano
- 1/3 cup dried basil
- ¼ cup pepper
- ¼ cup salt
- ¼ cup onion powder
- ¼ cup Dijon-style mustard
- 2 quarts red wine vinegar

Directions:

1. Take a large sized container and add olive oil, oregano, garlic powder, basil, salt, pepper, onion powder, Dijon-style mustard
2. Mix them well
3. Pour vinegar and mix vigorously yet again until the mix is well blended
4. Store tightly in a jar and use it whenever necessary

Nutrition:

- Calories: 123
- Fat: 4.7g
- Carbohydrates: 20g
- Protein: 2g

Breakfast Idea #11 - The Classical (Whole Foods) Baked French Fries

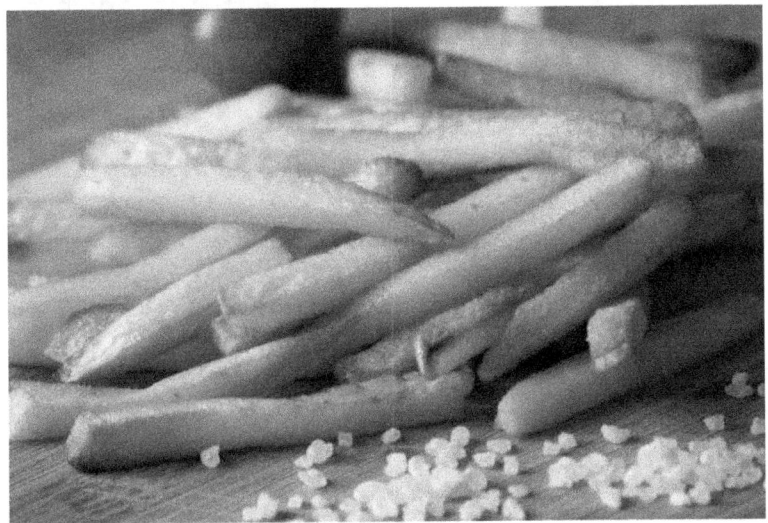

Prep Time: 5 minutes

Cooking Time: 45 minutes

Serving: 1

Ingredients:

- 1 large baking potato
- 1 tablespoon olive oil
- ½ a teaspoon paprika
- ½ a teaspoon garlic powder
- ½ a teaspoon chili powder
- ½ a teaspoon onion powder

Directions:

1. Pre-heat your oven to a temperature of 230 degrees Fahrenheit

2. Cut up your potato into wedges
3. Take a bowl and mix olive oil, garlic powder, paprika, chili powder, onion powder altogether
4. Coat up your potatoes with the spice/oil mix and place them on a fine baking sheet
5. Bake in your pre-heated oven for 45 minutes
6. Serve hot!

Nutrition:

- Calories: 357
- Fat: 14.1g
- Carbohydrates: 54.7g
- Protein: 5.4g

Breakfast Idea #12 - Delightfully Roasted Lemon Broccolis

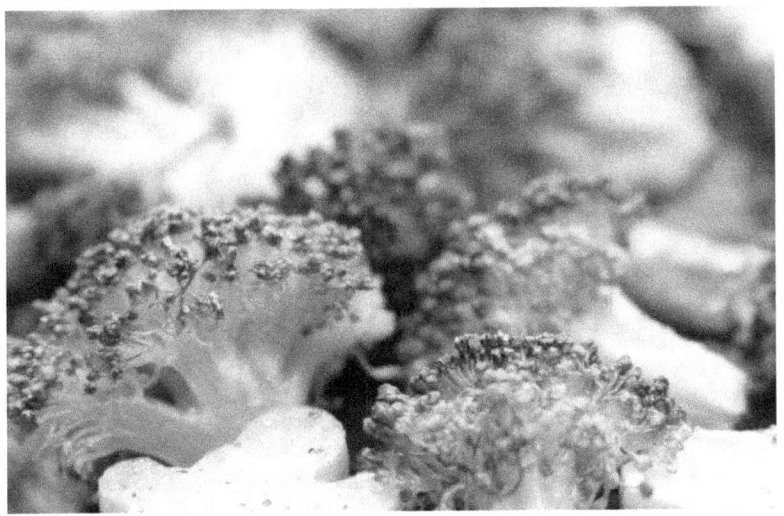

Prep Time: 10 minutes

Cooking Time: 15 minutes

Serving: 6

Ingredients:

- 2 heads broccoli separated into florets
- 2 teaspoon extra virgin olive oil
- 1 teaspoon sea salt
- ½ a teaspoon ground black pepper
- 1 minced garlic clove
- ½ a teaspoon lemon juice

Directions:

1. Pre-heat your oven to a temperature of 400 degrees Fahrenheit

2. Take a large sized bowl and add broccoli florets with some extra virgin olive oil, pepper, sea salt and garlic
3. Spread the broccoli out in a single even layer on a fine baking sheet
4. Bake in your pre-heated oven for about 15-20 minutes until the florets are soft enough so that they can be pierced with a fork
5. Squeeze lemon juice over them generously before serving
6. Enjoy!

Nutrition:

- Calories: 49
- Fat: 1.9g
- Carbohydrates: 7g
- Protein: 2.9g

Breakfast Idea #13 - The Whole Foods Guacamole

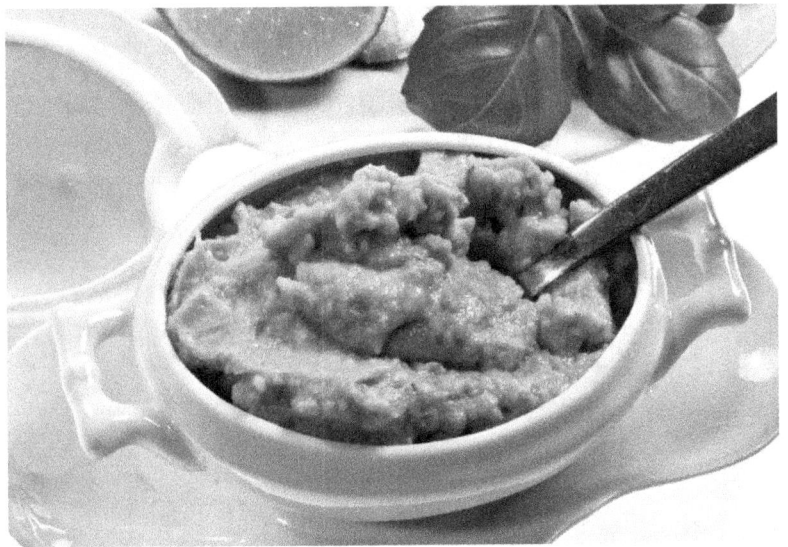

Prep Time: 10 minutes

Cooking Time: 0 minute

Serving: 4

Ingredients:

- 3 pieces peeled, mashed and pitted avocado
- 1 juiced lime
- 1 teaspoon salt
- ½ a cup diced onion
- 3 tablespoon chopped fresh cilantro
- 2 diced plum tomatoes
- 1 teaspoon minced garlic
- 1 pinch cayenne pepper

Directions:

1. Take a medium sized bowl and mash avocados, salt and lime juice
2. Stir in the tomatoes, onion, garlic and cilantro
3. Add cayenne pepper
4. Let it refrigerate for about an hour before serving
5. Serve chilled!

Nutrition:

- Calories: 262
- Fat: 22.2g
- Carbohydrates: 18g
- Protein: 3.7g

Breakfast Idea #14 - Eastern Chakchouka

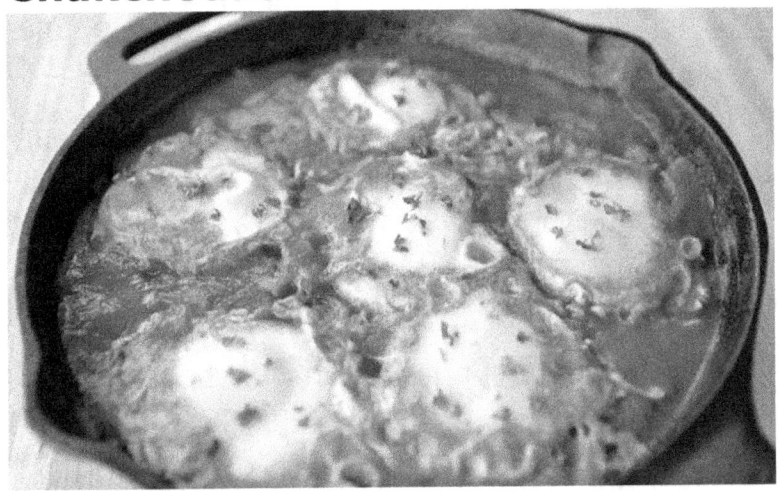

Prep Time: 20 minutes

Cooking Time: 20 minute

Serving: 4

Ingredients:

- 3 tablespoon olive oil
- 1 and a 1/3 cup chopped up onions
- 1 cup thinly sliced bell peppers
- 2 minced garlic cloves
- 2 and a ½ cups chopped tomatoes
- 1 teaspoon ground cumin
- 1 teaspoon paprika
- 1 teaspoon salt
- 1 hot chili pepper finely chopped and deseeded
- 4 eggs

Directions:

1. Take a skillet and put it over medium heat
2. Pour olive oil and heat it up
3. Stir in the onions, garlic and bell pepper and Sauté them for 5 minutes until soft and the onions are translucent
4. Take a bowl and combine cumin, tomatoes, salt, chili pepper and mix well
5. Pour the tomato mix into your skillet and keep stirring to combine gently
6. Simmer the mix uncovered for 10 minutes until the juices are cooked
7. Make four indentations in the mix using your finger and crack an egg into each of the indents
8. Cover the skillet and let it cook for another 5 minutes
9. Serve hot!

Nutrition:

- Calories: 209
- Fat: 15g
- Carbohydrates: 12g
- Protein: 7.8g

Breakfast Idea #15 - Feisty Collard Greens

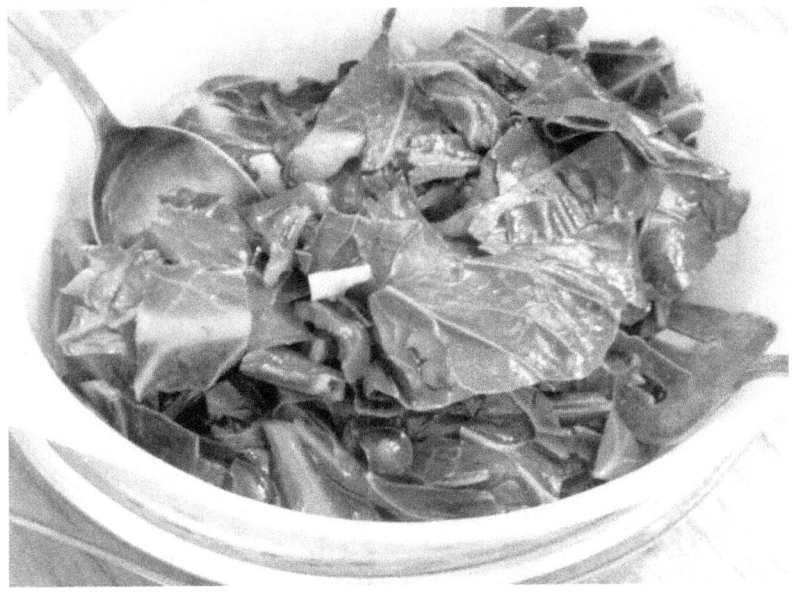

Prep Time: 10 minutes

Cooking Time: 1 hour

Serving: 6

Ingredients:

- 1 tablespoon olive oil
- 3 slices bacon
- 1 chopped up large onion
- 2 minced garlic cloves
- 1 teaspoon salt
- 3 cups chicken broth
- 1 pinch red pepper flakes
- 1 pound fresh collard greens cut up into 2 inch pieces

Directions:

1. Take a large pan and place it over medium-high heat
2. Pour oil and heat it up
3. Add bacon and cook it until crisp
4. Remove the bacon from the pan and crumble it
5. Return it to the pan
6. Add onion and keep cooking for 5 minutes until soft
7. Add garlic and cook until fragrant
8. Add collard greens and keep frying until they are starting to wilt
9. Pour the chicken broth and season the mix with some pepper, salt, and red pepper flakes
10. Lower down the heat to low and cover it up
11. Simmer for 45 minutes
12. Serve hot!

Nutrition:

- Calories: 127
- Fat: 9.2g
- Carbohydrates: 7.9g
- Protein: 4.4g

Breakfast Idea #16 - Spicy Mango and Avocado Salsa

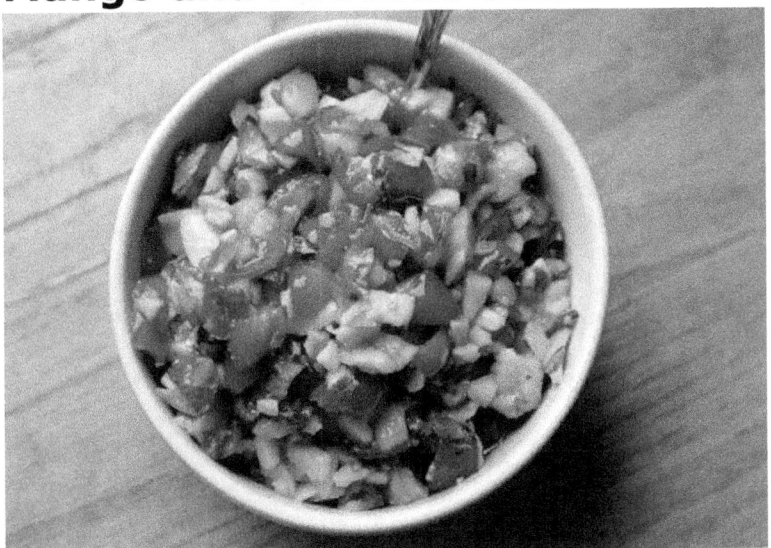

Prep Time: 10 minutes

Cooking Time: 30 minutes

Serving: 6

Ingredients:

- 1 peeled and deseeded mango (sliced)
- 1 peeled, pitted and diced avocado
- 4 medium sized diced tomatoes
- 1 deseeded and minced jalapeno pepper
- ½ a cup chopped up fresh cilantro
- 3 minced garlic cloves
- 1 teaspoon salt
- 2 tablespoon fresh lime juice
- ¼ cup chopped red onion
- 3 tablespoon olive oil

Directions:

1. Take a medium sized bowl
2. Combine avocado, mango, tomatoes, jalapeno, garlic, and cilantro
3. Stir in the salt, red onion, lime juice and olive oil
4. Place it in your fridge for 30 minutes before serving to fully blend the flavors
5. Use it as dipping for your favorite dipper

Nutrition:

- Calories: 158
- Fat: 12g
- Carbohydrates: 13g
- Protein: 1.9g

Breakfast Idea #17 - Tantalizing Garlic Salmon

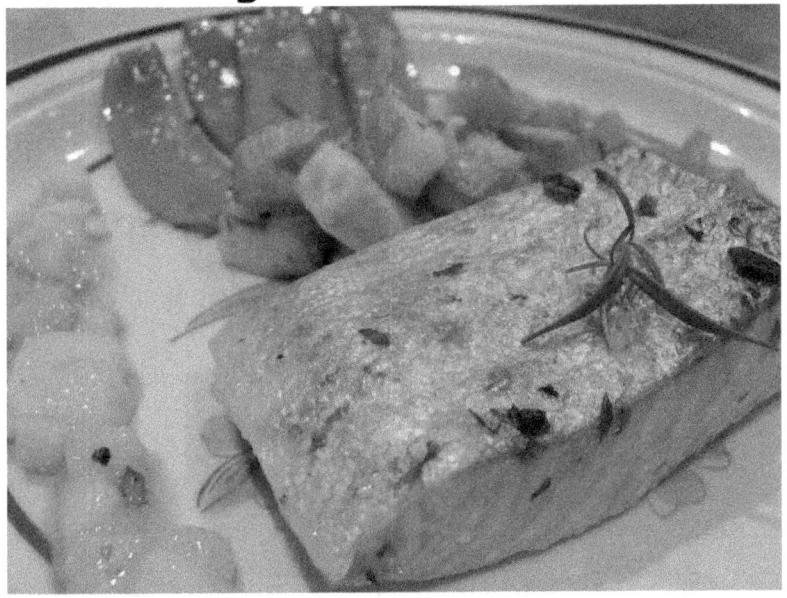

Prep Time: 15 minutes

Cooking Time: 25 minutes

Serving: 6

Ingredients:

- 1 and a ½ pound salmon fillet
- Salt as needed
- Pepper as needed
- 3 minced garlic cloves
- 1 chopped sprig fresh dill
- 5 lemon slices
- 5 fresh sprigs dill weed
- 2 chopped up green onions

Directions:

1. Pre-heat your oven to a temperature of 450 degrees Fahrenheit
2. Spray up two large pieces of aluminum cooking spray
3. Place the salmon fillets on top of your foil piece
4. Sprinkle some the salmon with some salt, garlic ,pepper and chopped dill
5. Arrange the lemon slices on top of your fillet
6. Place a sprig of dill on top of each of the lemon slices
7. Sprinkle chopped up scallions on top of the fillets
8. Cover the salmon with another piece of foil and pinch both of the foils together to seal it up
9. Place it on a baking sheet
10. Bake them in your pre-heated oven for 25 minutes
11. Make sure that the Salmon flakes off easily
12. Serve hot!

Nutrition:

- Calories: 169
- Fat: 6.78g
- Carbohydrates: 2.1g
- Protein: 24.5g

Breakfast Idea #18 - The Renowned Texas Salsa

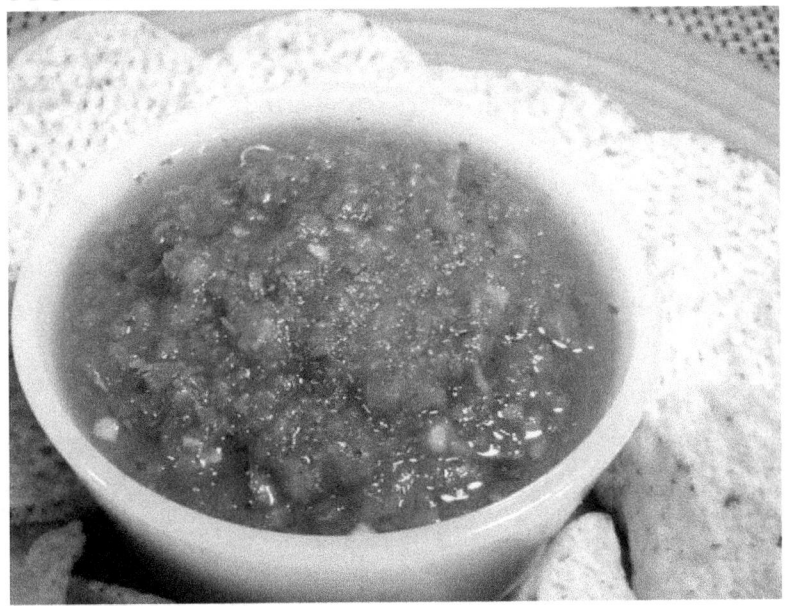

Prep Time: 10 minutes

Cooking Time: 30 minutes

Serving: 6

Ingredients:

- 2 cabs stewed tomatoes
- ½ finely diced onion
- 1 teaspoon minced garlic
- ½ a lime juice
- 1 teaspoon salt
- ¼ cup canned sliced green chills
- 3 tablespoon chopped fresh cilantro

Directions:

1. Open up the lid of your blender and add all of the listed ingredients in their specified portion
2. Blend them finely to your desired consistency
3. Use it as dipping for your favorite dipper

Nutrition:

- Calories: 158
- Fat: 12g
- Carbohydrates: 13g
- Protein: 1.9g

Breakfast Idea #19 - Healthy Cabbage Soup

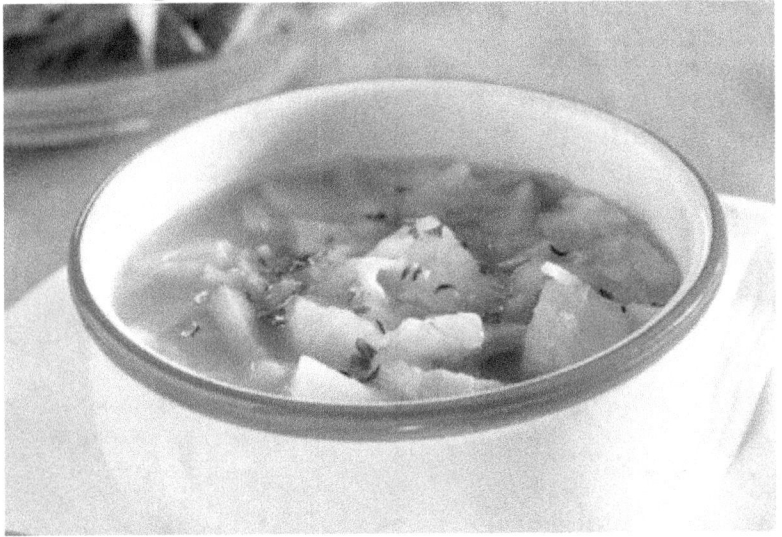

Prep Time: 30 minutes

Cooking Time: 45 minutes

Serving: 8

Ingredients:

- 3 tablespoon olive oil
- ½ chopped onion
- 2 chopped garlic cloves
- 2 quarts water
- 4 teaspoon chicken bouillon granules
- 1 teaspoon salt
- ½ teaspoon black pepper
- ½ cabbage head (chopped and cored)
- 14 ounce drained and diced tomatoes

Directions:

1. Take a large sized stockpot and pour olive oil over medium heat
2. Stir in the garlic and onion once the oil is hot and cook for 5 minutes
3. Stir in water, salt, bouillon, pepper
4. Bring the mix to a boil
5. Stir in the cabbage and simmer for another 10 minutes
6. Stir in the tomatoes and return it to boil once more
7. Simmer for 15-30 minutes
8. Make sure to keep stirring it from time to time
9. Serve!

Nutrition:

- Calories: 92
- Fat: 5.2g
- Carbohydrates: 8.6g
- Protein: 1.5g

Breakfast Idea #20 - The Perfect Good morning Boiled Egg

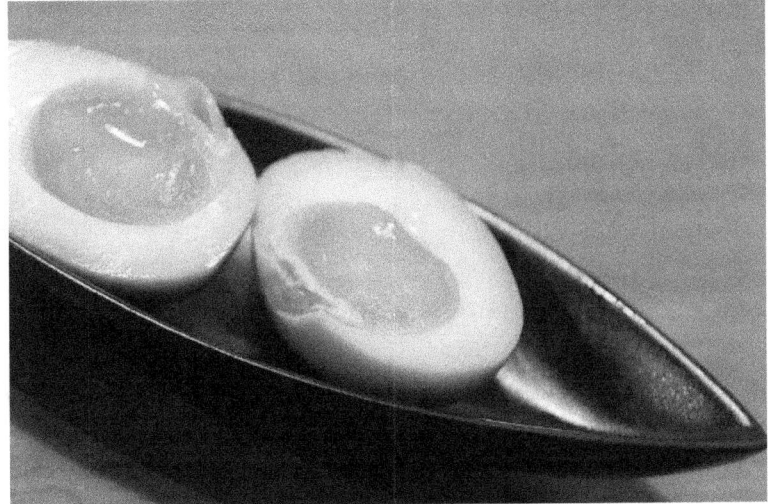

Prep Time: 5 minutes

Cooking Time: 20 minutes

Serving: 8

Ingredients:

- 1 tablespoon salt
- ¼ cup distilled white vinegar
- 6 cups water
- 8 eggs

Directions:

1. Take a large pot and combine salt, water, and vinegar
2. Bring the pot to a boil over high heat
3. Add one egg at a time

4. Lower down the heat to a gentle boil and cook for 14 minutes
5. Once done, remove the eggs from the water and place them in a container with cold water
6. Cool for 15 minutes
7. Store in your fridge for 1 week
8. Serve whenever desired

Nutrition:

- Calories: 72
- Fat: 5g
- Carbohydrates: 0.4g
- Protein: 6.3g

Breakfast Idea #21 - Tilapia (Grilled) With Mangos Salsa

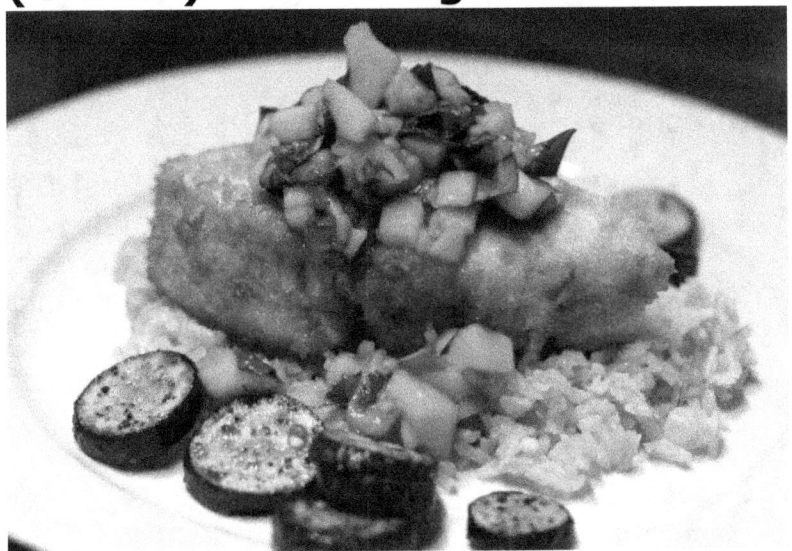

Prep Time: 45 minutes

Cooking Time: 10 minutes

Serving: 2

Ingredients:

- 1/3 cup extra-virgin olive oil
- 1 tablespoon minced fresh parsley
- 1 minced garlic clove
- 1 teaspoon dried basil
- 1 teaspoon ground black pepper
- ½ teaspoon salt
- 2 tilapia fillets
- 1 large, peeled, pitted and diced mango
- ½ diced red bell pepper
- 2 tablespoon minced red onion
- 1 tablespoon chopped up fresh cilantro

- 1 seeded and minced jalapeno pepper
- 2 tablespoon lime juice
- 1 tablespoon of lemon juice
- Salt as needed
- Pepper as needed

Directions:

1. Take a medium sized bowl and add the extra virgin olive oil, garlic, parsley, 1 teaspoon of pepper, ½ a teaspoon of salt
2. Mix them together and pour the mix into a resealable plastic bag
3. Add the tilapia fillets to the bag and coat it up with the marinade
4. Squeeze out the excess air and seal up the bag
5. Marinate the fish in your fridge for 1 hour
6. For the Mango Salsa, take a bowl and add mango, red onion, red bell pepper, cilantro, jalapeno pepper
7. Add the lime juice and 1 tablespoon of lemon juice
8. Toss it finely
9. Pre-heat your outdoor grill for medium-high heat settings and lightly oil up the grate
10. Remove the tilapia from the marinade and shake off the excess marinade
11. Discard the remaining marinade
12. Grill the fillets for 3-4 minutes per side until flaky
13. Serve with a topping of mango salsa

Nutrition:

- Calories: 634
- Fat: 40g
- Carbohydrates: 33g
- Protein: 36g

Breakfast Idea #22 - Easy Grilled Asparagus

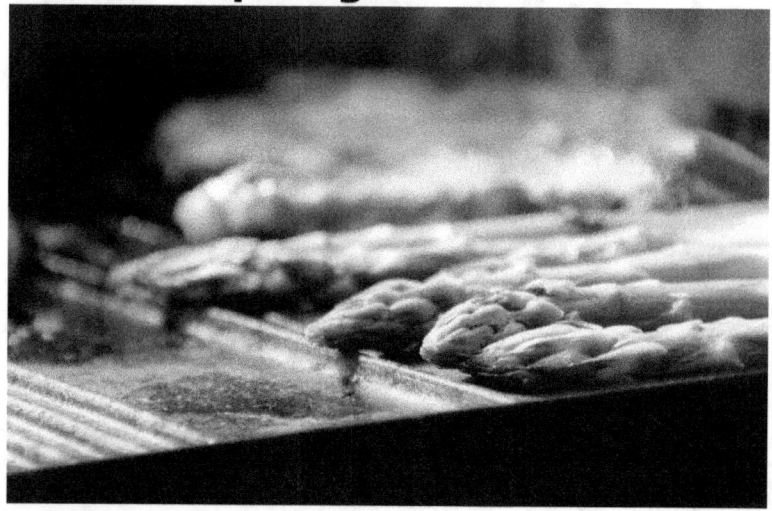

Prep Time: 15 minutes

Cooking Time: 3 minutes

Serving: 2

Ingredients:

- 1 pound trimmed asparagus
- 1 tablespoon olive oil
- Salt as needed
- Pepper as needed

Directions:

1. Pre-heat your grill for high-heat
2. Lightly coat up your asparagus spears with olive oil and season them with some pepper and salt
3. Grill them over high heat for 3 minutes
4. Serve hot!

Nutrition:

- Calories: 53
- Fat: 3.5g
- Carbohydrates: 4.4g
- Protein: 2.5g

Breakfast Idea #23 - Flavorful Unstuffed Cabbage Roll

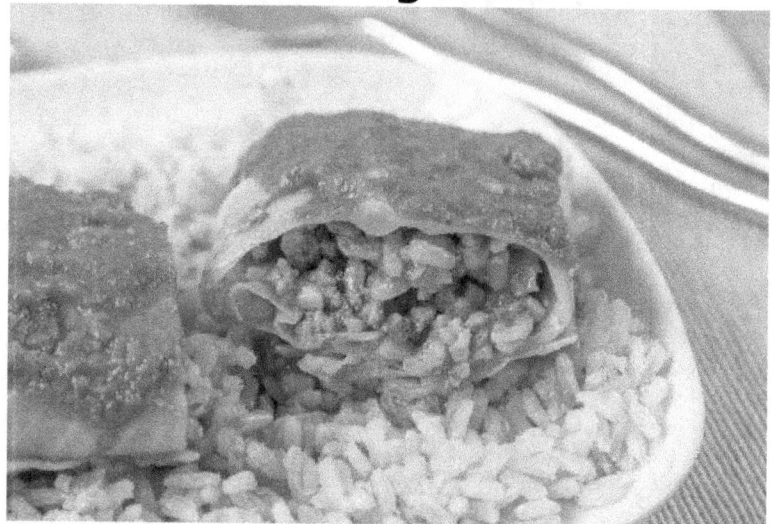

Prep Time: 20 minutes

Cooking Time: 35 minutes

Serving: 2

Ingredients:

- 2 pound ground beef
- 1 large sized chopped up onion
- 1 chopped up small head cabbage
- 2 cans diced tomatoes
- 8 ounce tomato sauce
- ½ cup water
- 2 minced garlic cloves
- 2 teaspoon salt
- 1 teaspoon ground black pepper

Directions:

1. Take a large sized skillet and place it over medium-high heat
2. Add the beef and onions and cook them for 5-7 minutes until nicely browned and crumbly
3. Drain and toss away the grease
4. Add tomatoes, cabbage, tomato sauce, garlic ,water, salt, pepper to the mix and bring it to a boil
5. Cover it up and reduce the heat
6. Simmer for 30 minutes until the cabbage is soft
7. Serve hot!

Nutrition:

- Calories: 398
- Fat: 23g
- Carbohydrates: 16.3g
- Protein: 28.5g

Breakfast Idea #24 - Energizing Mix Of Bacon, Garlic, Onion and Fried Cabbage

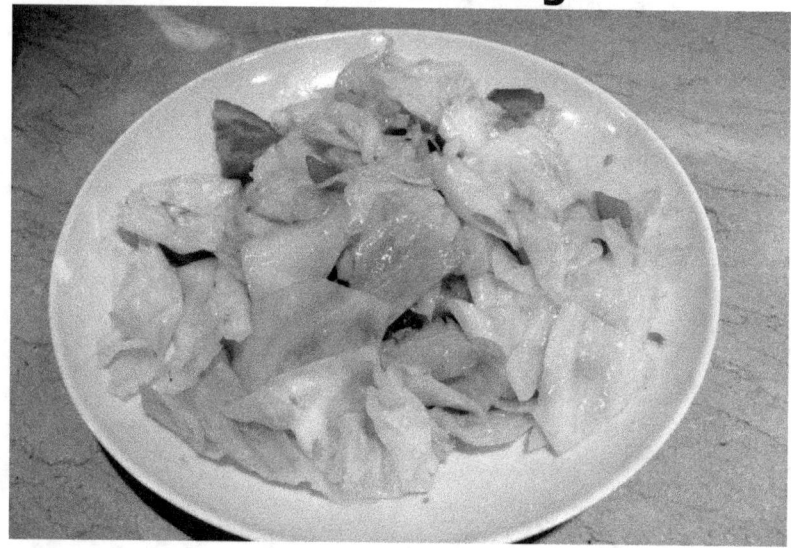

Prep Time: 15 minutes

Cooking Time: 60 minutes

Serving: 6

Ingredients:

- 6 chopped up bacon slices
- 1 diced large onion
- 2 minced garlic cloves
- 1 large cored and sliced cabbage head
- 1 tablespoon salt
- 1 teaspoon ground black pepper
- 1 teaspoon ground black pepper
- ½ teaspoon onion powder
- ½ teaspoon garlic powder

- 1/8 teaspoon paprika

Directions:

1. Take a large sized stock pot and add the bacon
2. Cook it over medium-high heat for 10 minutes until crispy and crumbly
3. Add garlic and onion
4. Cook and keep stirring It for 10 minutes to caramelize the onions
5. Stir in the cabbage and stir for yet another 10 minutes
6. Season with some onion powder, pepper, salt, paprika and garlic powder
7. Lower down the heat to low and cover it up
8. Simmer for 30 minutes, making sure to keep stirring it from time to time
9. Serve hot!

Nutrition:

- Calories: 194
- Fat: 12g
- Carbohydrates: 15g
- Protein: 6.4g

Breakfast Idea #25 - Green Beans With Sesame Seeds Spread Out

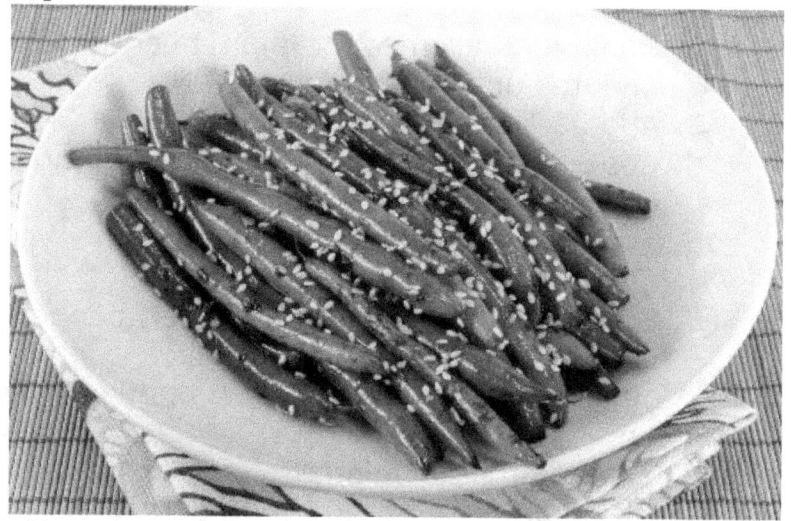

Prep Time: 5 minutes

Cooking Time: 25 minutes

Serving: 4

Ingredients:

- 1 tablespoon olive oil
- 1 tablespoon sesame seeds
- 1 pound fresh green beans cut up into 2 inch pieces
- ¼ cup chicken broth
- ¼ teaspoon salt
- Freshly ground black pepper

Directions:

1. Take a large sized skillet and place it over medium heat
2. Add oil and heat it up
3. Add sesame seeds
4. Once the seeds starts to darken, stir in the green beans
5. Keep cooking them until the beans turn bright green
6. Pour in the broth, pepper, and salt
7. Cover it up and cook for 10 minutes until the beans are crisp
8. Open up and cook for until the liquid is gone
9. Serve!

Nutrition:

- Calories: 78
- Fat: 4.6g
- Carbohydrates: 8.6g
- Protein: 2.5g

Breakfast Idea #26 - Peppers Stuffed With Vegetables and Turkey

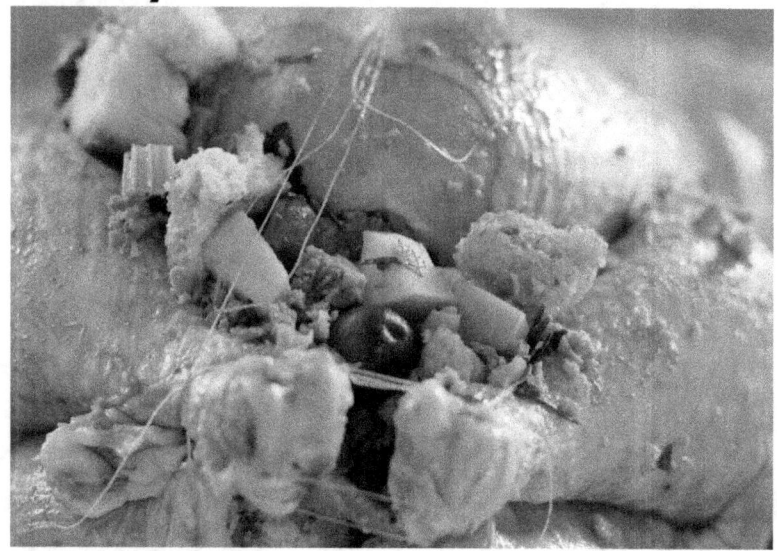

Prep Time: 20 minutes

Cooking Time: 30 minutes

Serving: 4

Ingredients:

- 4 green bell pepper with tops removed and deseeded
- 1 pound ground turkey
- 2 tablespoon of olive oil
- 1/2 chopped onion
- 1 cup sliced mushroom
- 1 chopped up zucchini
- ½ red chopped bell pepper
- ½ yellow chopped bell pepper

- 1 cup fresh spinach
- 14 ounce drained tomatoes
- 1 tablespoon tomato paste
- Italian seasoning
- Garlic as needed
- Salt as needed
- Pepper as needed

Directions:

1. Pre-heat your oven to a temperature of 350 degrees Fahrenheit
2. Wrap up your green bell peppers in aluminum foil and place them in your baking dish
3. Bake for about 15 minutes in your pre-heated oven
4. Remove the heat
5. Take a skillet and place it over medium heat
6. Cook the turkey until it is evenly browned
7. Set it aside
8. Pour oil to the skillet and heat the oil
9. Add onions, zucchini, mushrooms, red bell pepper, spinach, yellow bell pepper and cook them until soft
10. Return the turkey to the skillet
11. Mix in the tomatoes, tomato paste and season with garlic powder, Italian seasoning, pepper and salt
12. Stuff the green peppers with mixture made in the skillet
13. Return the peppers to the oven and cook for another 15 minutes

14.   Serve hot!

Nutrition:

- Calories: 280
- Fat: 15g
- Carbohydrates: 10.2g
- Protein: 25g

Breakfast Idea #27 - Not Too Fancy Butternut Squash Roast

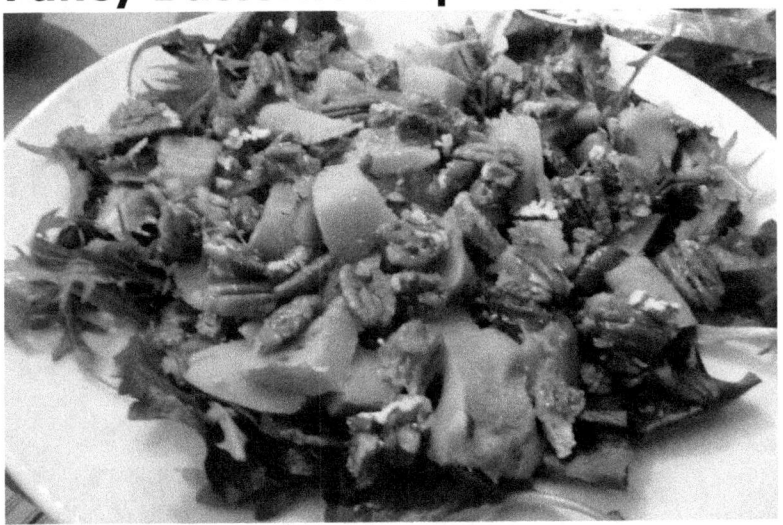

Prep Time: 15 minutes

Cooking Time: 25 minutes

Serving: 4

Ingredients:

- 1 piece butternut squash
- 2 tablespoon olive oil
- 2 mince garlic cloves
- Salt as needed
- Pepper as needed

Directions:

1. Pre-heat your oven to a temperature of 400 degrees Fahrenheit
2. Toss your butternut squash with garlic and olive oil in a large sized bowl

3. Season them with some black pepper and salt
4. Arrange the coated squash on a baking sheet
5. Roast them in a pre-heated oven for 25-30 minutes until the squash is tender and slightly browned

Nutrition:

- Calories: 177
- Fat: 7g
- Carbohydrates: 30g
- Protein: 2.6g

Breakfast Idea #28 - Fully Smothered Green Beans

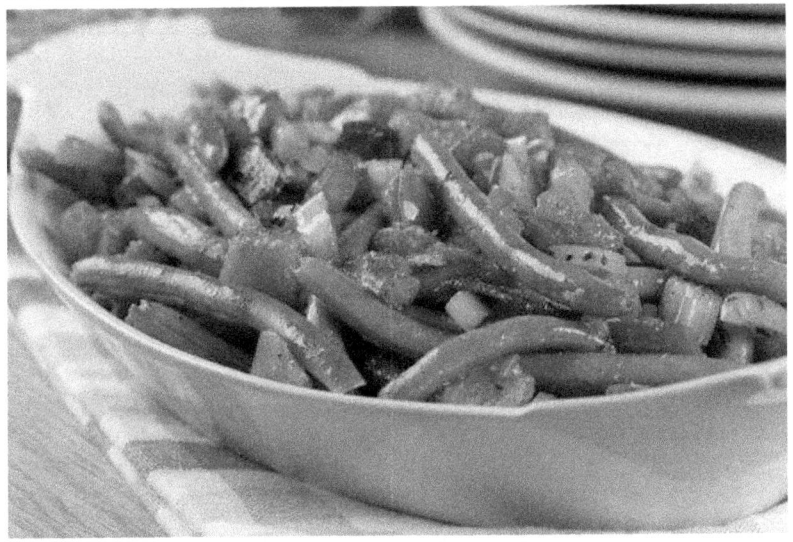

Prep Time: 15 minutes

Cooking Time: 25 minutes

Serving: 6

Ingredients:

- 6 thick slices chopped bacon
- ½ cup minced onion
- 1 teaspoon minced garlic
- 1 pound trimmed fresh green beans
- 1 cup water
- 1/8 teaspoon salt
- 1 pinch ground black pepper

Directions:

1. Take a large sized deep skillet

2. Add the bacon and cook it over medium-high heat until the fat slowly begins to render
3. Stir in the garlic, onions and cook for another 1 minute
4. Add water and the beans and let them cook until the water has been evaporated and the beans are soft
5. Add some more water to cook for some added time if beans not soft by the end of the evaporation
6. Season with pepper and salt
7. Serve!

Nutrition:

- Calories: 97
- Fat: 5.4g
- Carbohydrates: 7g
- Protein: 6.2g

Breakfast Idea #29 - Special Kielbasa With Potatoes and Peppers

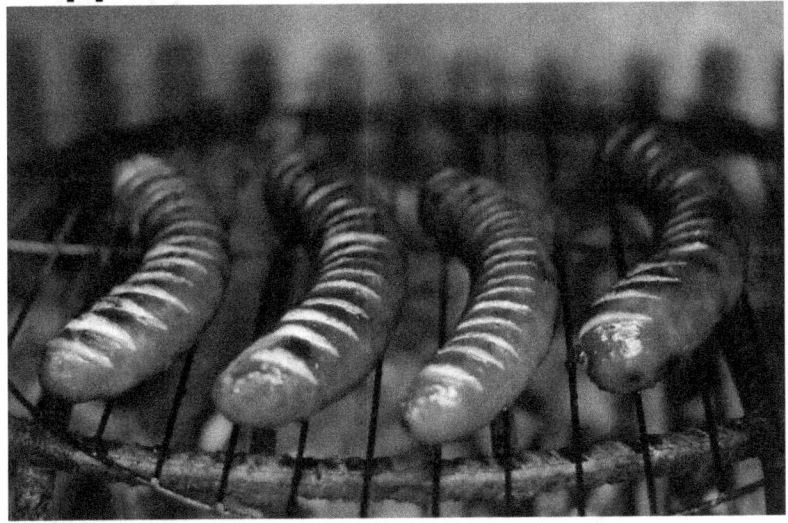

Prep Time: 10 minutes

Cooking Time: 30 minutes

Serving: 6

Ingredients:

- 1 tablespoon vegetable oil
- 15 ounce package smoked kielbasa sausage all diced up
- 6 medium sized diced red potatoes
- 1 sliced red bell pepper
- 1 sliced yellow bell pepper

Directions:

1. Take a saucepan over medium heat and heat up some oil
2. Place the sausages and potatoes in the pan
3. Cover it up and cook for 25 minutes, makings sure to keep stirring it from time to time until the potatoes are soft
4. Add the yellow and red peppers into the pan
5. Keep cooking for another 5 minutes until the peppers are soft
6. Serve!

Nutrition:

- Calories: 404
- Fat: 23g
- Carbohydrates: 36g
- Protein: 13g

Breakfast Idea #30 - Cute And Crispy Fish Fillets

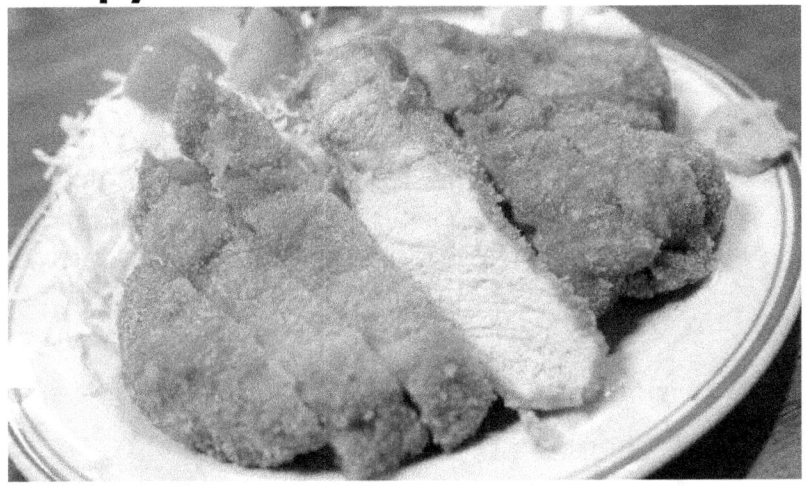

Prep Time: 10 minutes

Cooking Time: 10 minutes

Serving: 4

Ingredients:

- 1 egg
- 2 tablespoon prepared yellow mustard
- 1/2 teaspoon salt
- 1 and ½ cup instant mashed potato flakes
- ¼ cup olive oil
- 6 ounce fillets

Directions:

1. Take a shallow dish and whisk in the eggs, salt, and mustard

2. Keep it on the side
3. Add potato flakes in another shallow dish
4. Take a large sized heavy skillet and place it over medium-high heat
5. Heat up oil
6. Dip the fish fillets in the mixture
7. Dredge the fillets in your potato flakes and make sure to coat up the fish nicely
8. Fry the fillets for 3-4 minutes in oil for each of the sides until la golden brown texture is seen
9. Serve hot!

Nutrition:

- Calories: 391
- Fat: 18g
- Carbohydrates: 26g
- Protein: 30g

Chapter 2: 30 Lunch Ideas

Lunch Idea #1 - Fine Lemon Rosemary Salmon

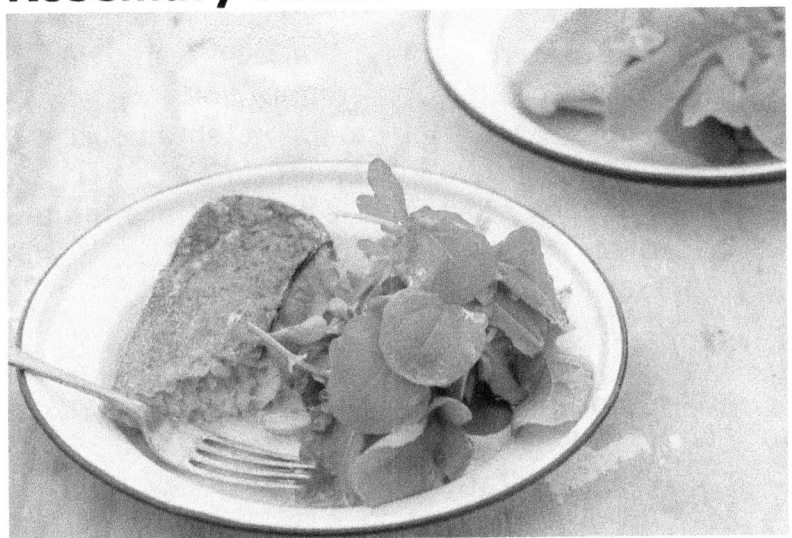

Prep Time: 10 minutes

Cooking Time: 20 minutes

Serving: 2

Ingredients:

- 1 thinly sliced lemon
- 4 sprigs rosemary
- 2 de-boned and skinned salmon fillets
- Coarse salt as needed
- 1 tablespoon olive oil

Directions:

1. Pre-heat your oven to a temperature of 400 degrees Fahrenheit
2. Take a baking dish and arrange half of your lemon slices in a single layer
3. Create a layer using your sprigs of rosemary and top them up with your fillets
4. Sprinkle the salmon with salt and make another layer of rosemary sprigs
5. Top up with the remaining lemon slices
6. Drizzle some olive oil on top
7. Bake for 20 minutes in your pre-heated oven (Check for flaky texture)
8. Serve hot!

Nutrition:

- Calories: 257
- Fat: 18g
- Carbohydrates: 6.1g
- Protein: 20.5g

Lunch Idea #2 - Chicken Breast Cooked With A Herbal Basting Sauce

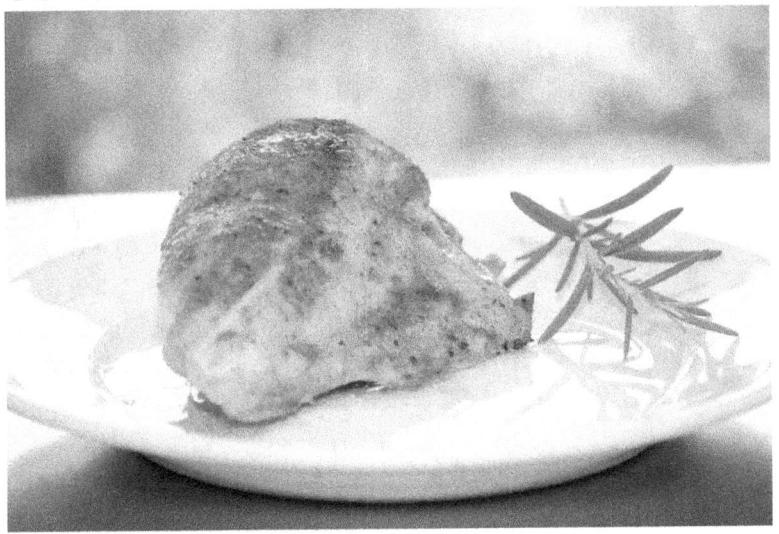

Prep Time: 10 minutes

Cooking Time: 20 minutes

Serving: 2

Ingredients:

- 3 tablespoon olive oil
- 1 tablespoon minced onion
- 1 clove crushed garlic
- 1 teaspoon dried thyme
- ½ teaspoon crushed dried rosemary
- ¼ teaspoon ground sage
- ¼ teaspoon dried marjoram
- ½ teaspoon salt
- ½ teaspoon ground black pepper
- 1/8 teaspoon hot pepper sauce

- 4 bone-in chicken breast halves
- 1 and ½ teaspoon chopped up fresh parsley

Directions:

1. Pre-heat your oven to a temperature of 425 degrees Fahrenheit
2. Take a bowl and add the olive oil, garlic, onion, thyme, sage, rosemary, pepper, salt and hot pepper sauce and combine them gently to create your basting sauce
3. Turn the chicken breast in the sauce and coat it up evenly
4. Place the marinated chicken in a shallow baking dish with the skin side facing up
5. Roast the chicken at 425 degrees Fahrenheit for 35-25 minutes, making sure to keep basting it from time to time using the pan drippings
6. Remove it to a warm platter
7. Spoon the pan juices over them and sprinkle some fresh parsley
8. Enjoy!

Nutrition:

- Calories: 391
- Fat: 21.9g
- Carbohydrates: 1.1g
- Protein: 45.1g

Lunch Idea #3 - Grilled Up Portobello Mushrooms

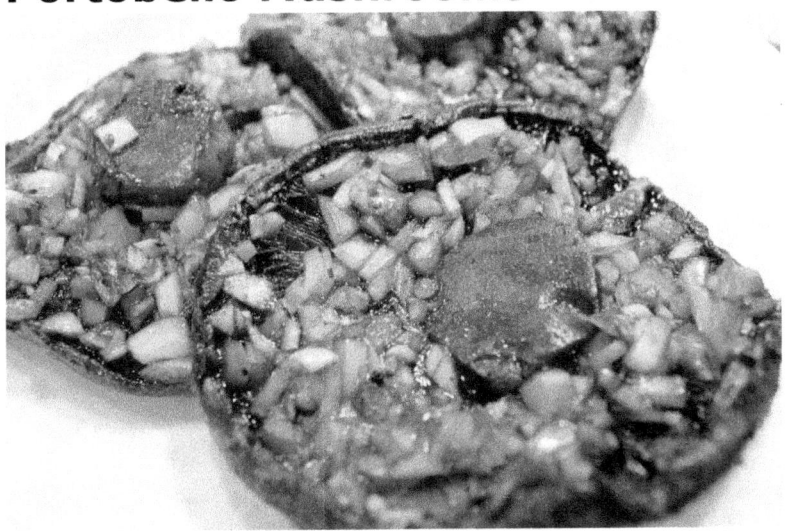

Prep Time: 10 minutes

Cooking Time: 10 minutes

Serving: 2

Ingredients:

- 3 Portobello mushrooms
- ¼ cup canola oil
- 3 tablespoon chopped onion
- 4 minced clove garlic
- 4 tablespoon balsamic vinegar

Directions:

1. Clean up the mushrooms finely and remove the stems
2. Keep it on the side for later use

3. Place the caps on a plate with the gills siding upward
4. Take a small sized bowl and combine onion, oil, vinegar and garlic
5. Pour mix evenly all over your mushroom caps and let it stand for about an hour
6. Grill them over a hot grill for 10 minutes and serve hot!

Nutrition:

- Calories: 217
- Fat: 19g
- Carbohydrates: 11g
- Protein: 3.2g

Lunch Idea #4 - Wonderful Artichokes And Sun Dried Tomatoes

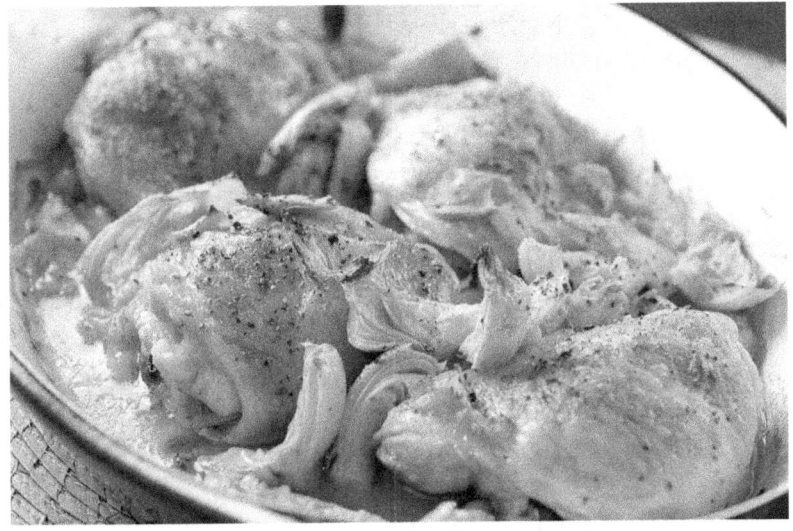

Prep Time: 10 minutes

Cooking Time: 25 minutes

Serving: 4

Ingredients:

- 4 boneless chicken breasts (skinless)
- Salt as needed
- Pepper as needed
- 2 teaspoon olive oil
- 14 ounce diced tomatoes, green peppers, and onions
- ¼ cup sun dried tomato pesto
- 14 ounce artichoke hearts (Drained and quartered)

Directions:

1. Season up both sides of your chicken breasts with pepper and salt
2. Take a large sized skillet and heat it over medium-high heat
3. Add oil and heat it up
4. Place your chicken in a skillet and cook, making sure to turn once to brown both sides of the chicken
5. Remove the chicken from your pan and keep it aside
6. Pour tomatoes into the pan and cook for another minute, make sure to stir it constantly
7. Stir in the artichokes, pesto and return it to your pan
8. Cover it up and reduce the heat to a medium
9. Simmer for another 5-10 minutes
10.   Serve hot!

Nutrition:

- Calories: 228
- Fat: 6.5g
- Carbohydrates: 11.4g
- Protein: 30g

Lunch Idea #5 - Fresh Avocado and Fennel Salad

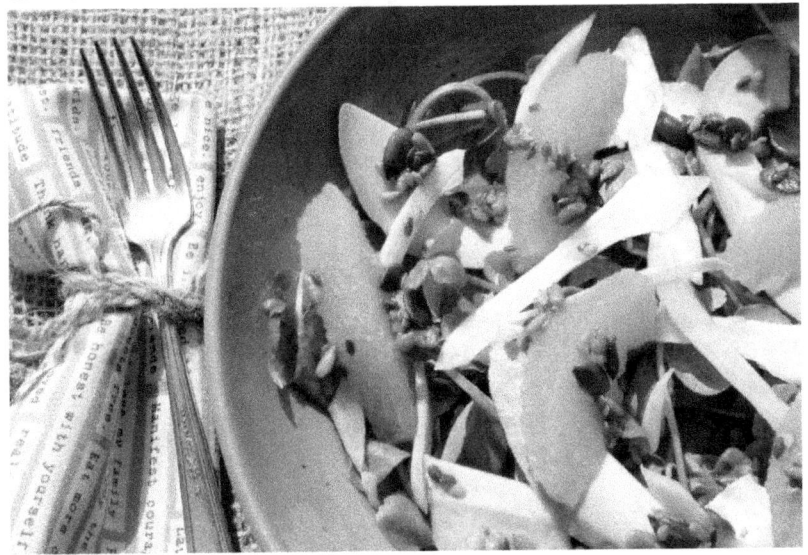

Prep Time: 10 minutes

Cooking Time: 0 minute

Serving: 4

Ingredients:

- 3 thinly sliced fennel bulbs
- 1 peeled, cubed and pitted avocado
- 2 tablespoon extra virgin olive oil
- 1 teaspoon ground nutmeg
- Salt as needed

Directions:

1. Take a salad bowl and add the avocado and fennel

2. Stir in some oil, salt, nutmeg and mix them all well
3. Serve!

Nutrition:

- Calories: 130
- Fat: 8.4g
- Carbohydrates: 13.8g
- Protein: 2.4g

Lunch Idea #6 - Rinsed Acapulco Chicken

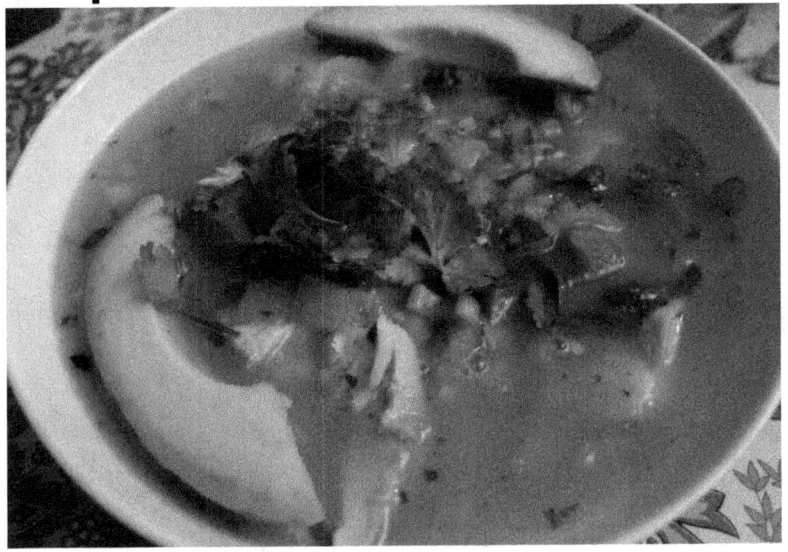

Prep Time: 10 minutes

Cooking Time: 15 minutes

Serving: 2

Ingredients:

- 2 skinless and boneless (halved) chicken breasts cut up into bite sized pieces
- 1 tablespoon divide chili powder
- Salt as needed
- Pepper as needed
- 1 tablespoon olive oil
- 1 cup chopped up green bell pepper
- ½ cup chopped onion
- 2 jalapeno peppers minced and seeded
- 1 large sized tomato cut up into chunks
- 10 drops hot pepper sauce

Directions:

1. Season up the chicken with ½ a tablespoon of chili powder, pepper, and salt
2. Take a large sized skillet and place it over medium-high heat
3. Heat up the oil and Sauté your seasoned chicken for 4 minutes
4. Remove them from the skillet using a slotted spoon and keep them warm
5. In the same skillet, stir-fry your onion and bell pepper until they are tender
6. Add the tomatoes, jalapeno peppers, hot pepper sauce and ½ a tablespoon of chili powder
7. Cook for another 3-5 minutes, making sure to keep stirring them
8. Add the chicken then and stir-fry for another 2 minutes
9. Serve hot!

Nutrition:

- Calories: 333
- Fat: 13g
- Carbohydrates: 23g
- Protein: 30g

Lunch Idea #7 - The Genuine American Roast Beef

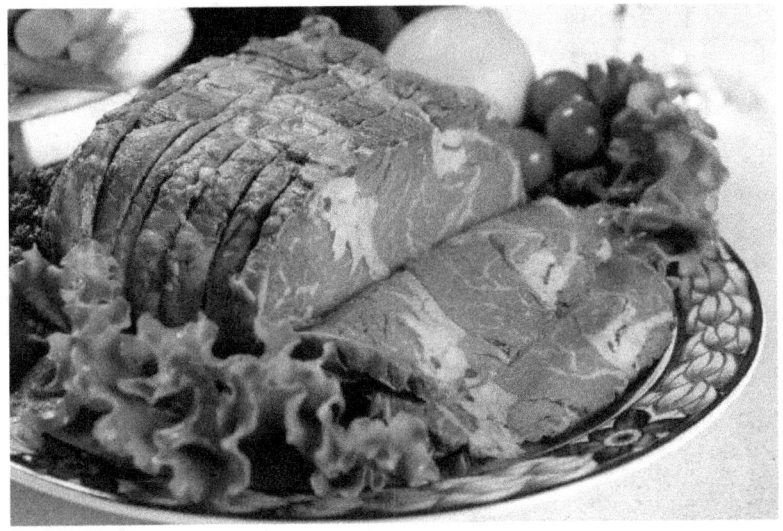

Prep Time: 5 minutes

Cooking Time: 60 minutes

Serving: 6

Ingredients:

- 3 pounds beef eye round roast
- ½ teaspoon kosher salt
- ½ teaspoon garlic powder
- ¼ teaspoon freshly ground black pepper

Directions:

1. Pre-heat your oven to a temperature of 375 degrees Fahrenheit
2. Tie up the roast at 3-inch intervals using a cotton twine

3. Place the tied roast in your twine and season with garlic powder, salt, and pepper
4. Add some extra seasoning for added flavor
5. Roast it in your oven for 60 minutes
6. Remove them from the oven once done and cover it loosely with a foil
7. Let it rest for 20 minutes and serve!

Nutrition:

- Calories: 484
- Fat: 32g
- Carbohydrates: 0.2g
- Protein: 44g

Lunch Idea #8 - The Perfect Ethiopian Cabbage Dish

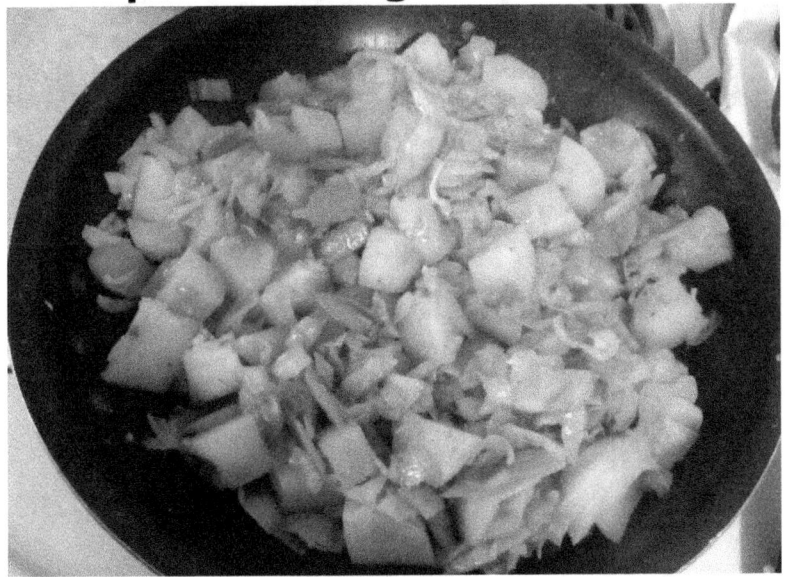

Prep Time: 25 minutes

Cooking Time: 40 minutes

Serving: 5

Ingredients:

- ½ cup olive oil
- 4 thinly sliced carrots
- 1 thinly sliced onion
- 1 teaspoon tea salt
- ½ teaspoon ground black pepper
- ½ teaspoon ground cumin
- ¼ teaspoon ground black pepper
- ½ teaspoon ground cumin
- ¼ teaspoon ground turmeric
- ½ shredded cabbage head

- 5 potatoes peeled and cut up into 1-inch cubes

Directions:

1. Take a skillet and heat up some oil over medium heat
2. Toss in the carrots and onion and Sauté them for about 5 minutes
3. Stir in the pepper, salt, cumin, turmeric, cabbage and cook for an extra 15-20 minutes
4. Add the potatoes then
5. Cover it up and lower down the heat to medium-low levels
6. Cook for another 20-30 minutes until the potatoes are tender
7. Serve hot

Nutrition:

- Calories: 428
- Fat: 22.2g
- Carbohydrates: 54.1g
- Protein: 6.9g

Lunch Idea #9 - Cool Steam Fish with Lemon Dashes

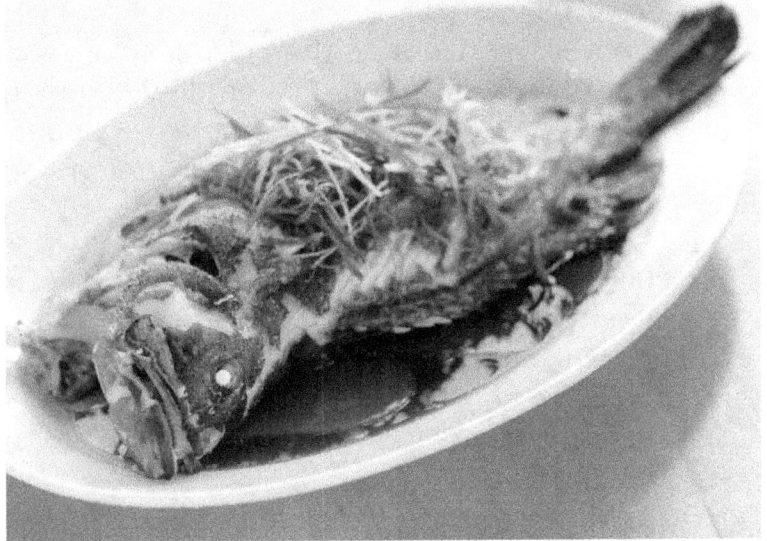

Prep Time: 25 minutes

Cooking Time: 40 minutes

Serving: 5

Ingredients:

- 6 ounce halibut fillets
- 1 tablespoon dried dill weed
- 1 tablespoon onion powder
- 2 teaspoon dried parsley
- ¼ teaspoon paprika
- 1 pinch salt
- 1 pinch lemon pepper
- 1 pinch garlic powder
- 2 tablespoon lemon juice

Directions:

1. Pre-heat your oven to a temperature of 375 degrees Fahrenheit
2. Cut up a foil into 6 squares in the size of your fillets
3. Center the fillets on the cut foil squares
4. Sprinkle dill weed, parsley, onion powder, paprika, lemon pepper, seasoned salt and garlic powder on top of the fillets
5. Sprinkle some lemon juice on top of each fillet
6. Fold the foil over your fillets and make a pocket and fold from edge to edge in order to seal it
7. Place the sealed packets on top of a baking sheet
8. Bake in your oven for about 30 minutes until the fish flakes come off easily using a fork
9. Serve hot!

Nutrition:

- Calories: 142
- Fat: 1.1g
- Carbohydrates: 1.9g
- Protein: 29.7g

Lunch Idea #10 - The Basic (Juicy) BBQ Ribs

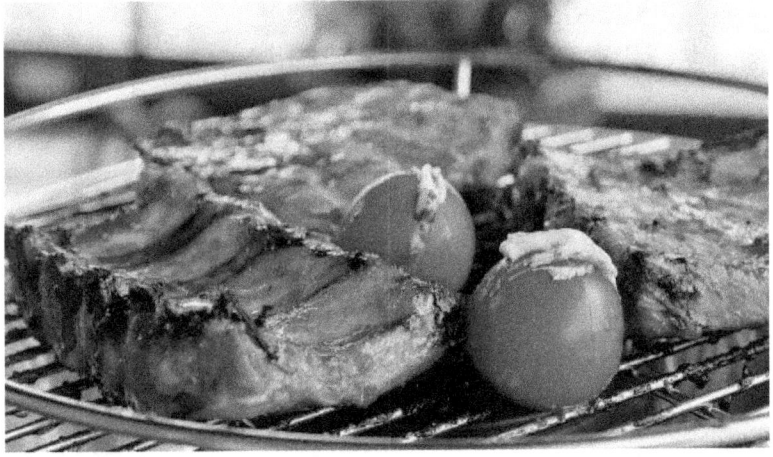

Prep Time: 30 minutes

Cooking Time: 1 Hour 30 minutes

Serving: 4

Ingredients:

- 2 and ½ pound country style pork ribs
- 1 tablespoon garlic powder
- 1 teaspoon ground black pepper
- 2 tablespoon salt
- 1 cup BBQ sauce

Directions:

1. Take a large sized pot and add the ribs
2. Fill it up with enough water to cover the ribs
3. Season with black pepper, garlic powder, salt

4. Bring the water to a boil and cook the ribs until they are soft
5. Pre-heat your oven to a temperature of 325 degrees Fahrenheit
6. Remove the ribs from your pot and add them to a 9x13 inch baking dish
7. Pour the BBQ sauce over the ribs
8. Cover the dish with aluminum foil
9. Bake them in your pre-heated oven for about 1 to 1 and a ½ hours
10. Make sure to check that the internal temperature has reached 160 degrees Fahrenheit
11. Serve!

Nutrition:

- Calories: 441
- Fat: 22.2g
- Carbohydrates: 24.5g
- Protein: 33.3g

Lunch Idea #11 - Fancy Salmon Burgers With Avocado Mix

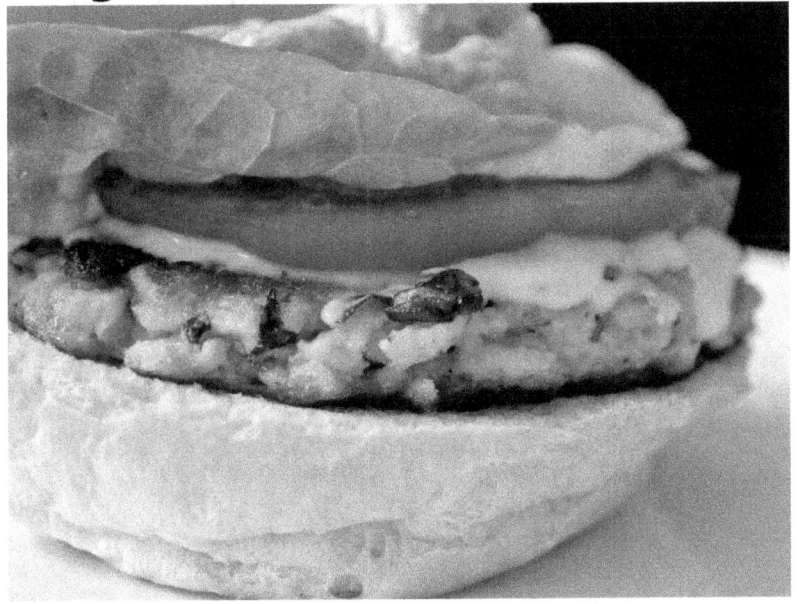

Prep Time: 20 minutes

Cooking Time: 8 minutes

Serving: 4

Ingredients:

For Patty

- 1 pound salmon fillet
- ½ cup almond meal
- 1 piece egg
- 2 chopped up green onions
- ½ seeded and chopped poblano pepper
- 1 tablespoon fresh lime juice
- ½ teaspoon salt
- ¼ teaspoon pepper

For Avocado Salsa

- 1 large sized ripe and peeled avocado
- ½ of a seeded and chopped poblano pepper
- 2 pieces of green onions
- ¼ teaspoon of salt
- ¼ teaspoon of pepper
- ¼ teaspoon of salt

Directions:

1. Finely skin and chop up your Salmon fillet
2. Take a large sized bowl and add the fillets to that bowl
3. Add poblano, almond meal, egg, lime juice, pepper and salt to the bowl
4. Heat up your indoor grill to a medium-high level
5. Cook it for about 4 minutes on each of the sides to make sure that it is thoroughly cooked
6. For the salad, take a medium sized bowl and mix all of the listed ingredients
7. Top up your burgers with the salsa mix and serve with your preferred bun

Nutrition:

- Calories: 353
- Fat: 22.9g
- Carbohydrates: 12.4g
- Protein: 25.4g

Lunch Idea #12 - Baby Back Ribs With BBQ Sauce

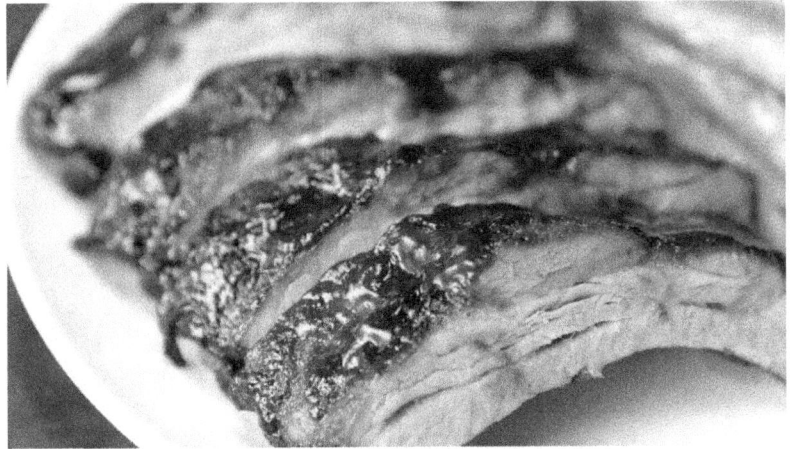

Prep Time: 8 hours

Cooking Time: 2 hours 30 minutes

Serving: 4

Ingredients:

- 2 pound organic baby back pork ribs
- 18 ounce barbecue sauce

Directions:

1. Gently tear off 4 pieces off aluminum foil that should be big enough to completely enclose the portions of your ribs
2. Spray each of the piece of foil with vegetable cooking spray
3. Brush up the ribs generously with BBQ sauce and place the ribs on top of their respective foils

4. Wrap them tightly and let them refrigerate for at least 8 hours or overnight
5. Pre-heat your oven to a temperature of 300 degrees Fahrenheit
6. Bake the ribs for 2 and ½ hours
7. Remove them from the foil and add some more sauce if desired
8. Serve hot!

Nutrition:

- Calories: 698
- Fat: 37.4g
- Carbohydrates: 45.7g
- Protein: 43.2g

Lunch Idea #13 - Lightly Braised Balsamic Chicken

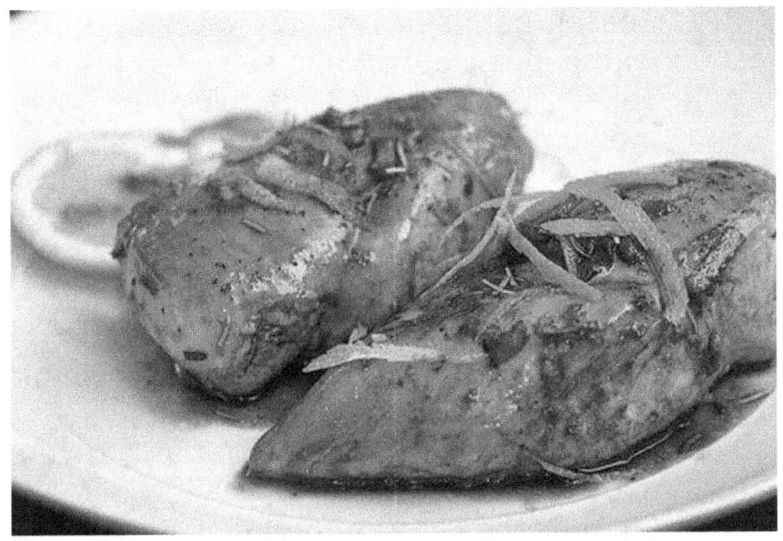

Prep Time: 10 minutes

Cooking Time: 25 minutes

Serving: 6

Ingredients:

- 6 boneless, skinless chicken breast halves
- 1 teaspoon garlic salt
- Ground black pepper as needed
- 2 tablespoon olive oil
- 1 thinly sliced onion
- 1 can diced tomatoes
- ½ cup balsamic vinegar
- 1 teaspoon dried basil
- 1 teaspoon dried oregano
- 1 teaspoon dried rosemary

- ½ teaspoon dried thyme

Directions:

1. Season both sides of your chicken breast with pepper, garlic, and salt
2. Take a skill and heat olive oil over medium heat
3. Cook the seasoned chicken breasts for 3-4 minutes per side until they are nicely browned
4. Add onions and keep cooking for another 3-4 minutes to brown them
5. Pour the diced up tomatoes, balsamic vinegar over chicken
6. Season with some oregano, basil, thyme and rosemary
7. Simmer the chicken for 15 minutes until it is no longer pink and the juice run clear
8. Use an instant-read thermometer to check the internal temperature which should read 165 degrees Fahrenheit
9. Serve

Nutrition:

- Calories: 196
- Fat: 7g
- Carbohydrates: 7.6g
- Protein: 23.8g

Lunch Idea #14 - Mouthwatering Grilled Shrimp

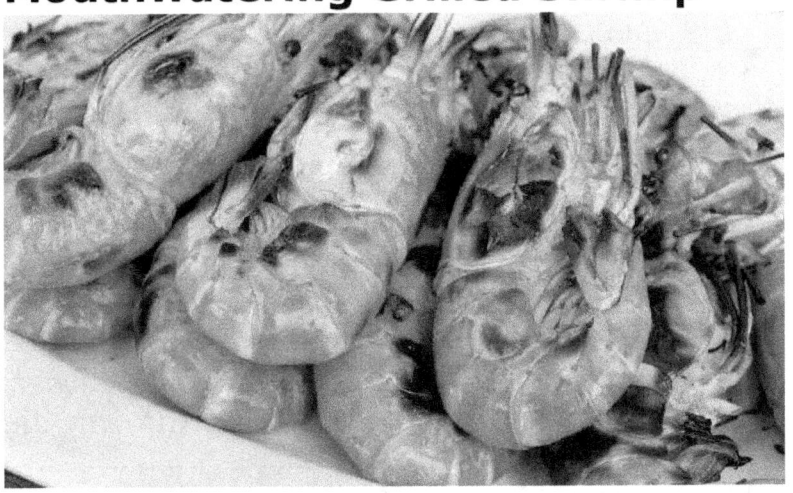

Prep Time: 30 minutes

Cooking Time: 10 minutes

Serving: 6

Ingredients:

- 1 juiced lemon juice
- 2 tablespoon hot pepper sauce
- 3 minced garlic cloves
- 1 tablespoon tomato paste
- 2 teaspoon dried oregano
- 1 teaspoon salt
- 1 teaspoon ground black pepper
- 2 pound large peeled and deveined shrimps
- Skewers

Directions:

1. Take a mixing bowl and add olive oil, lemon juice, parsley, hot sauce, tomato paste, garlic, salt, oregano and black pepper
2. Mix them well
3. Keep a small amount on the side for later basting
4. Pour the rest of the marinade into a resealable bag alongside the shrimp
5. Seal it up and marinate it in your fridge for 2 hours
6. Pre-heat your over medium-low heat
7. Thread the shrimps onto your skewer, making sure to pierce them through the tail to the head
8. Discard the marinade
9. Gently oil the grill grate
10. Cook the shrimp for 5 minutes per side, making sure to keep basting it from time to time using the reserved marinade
11. Serve

Nutrition:

- Calories: 447
- Fat: 37g
- Carbohydrates: 3.7g
- Protein: 25.3g

Lunch Idea #15 - Brussels sprouts Roast

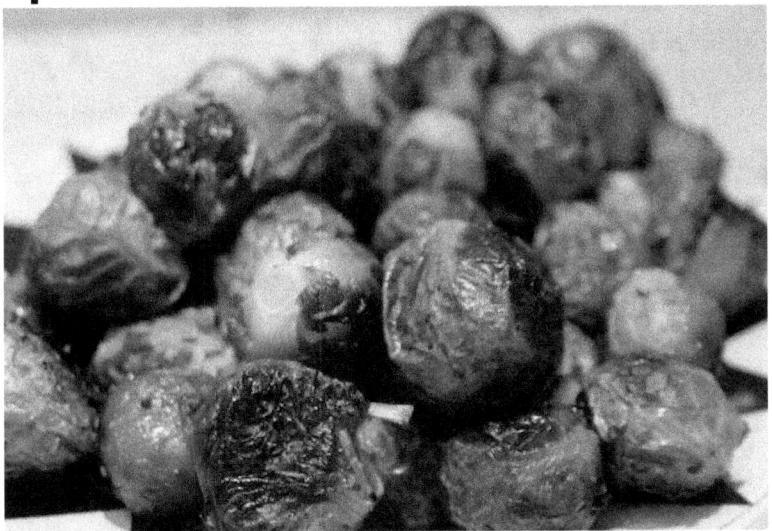

Prep Time: 15 minutes

Cooking Time: 45 minutes

Serving: 6

Ingredients:

- 1 and ½ pound Brussels sprouts with ends trimmed up
- 3 tablespoon olive oil
- 1 teaspoon kosher salt
- ½ teaspoon finely ground black pepper

Directions:

1. Pre-heat your oven to a temperature of 400 degrees Fahrenheit

2. Place your trimmed Brussels sprouts, kosher salt, olive oil and pepper in a large re-sealable bag
3. Seal it tightly and shake finely to coat it up
4. Pour in onto a baking sheet and place it on the center rack of your oven
5. Roast it in your pre-heated oven for about 45 minutes, making sure to shake the tray after every 5 minutes
6. Lower down the heat if you notice burning
7. Once the sprouts show a dark brown texture, adjust the seasoning with some salt and serve hot

Nutrition:

- Calories: 104
- Fat: 7.3g
- Carbohydrates: 10g
- Protein: 2.9g

Lunch Idea #16 - Balsamic Pork Loin Roast

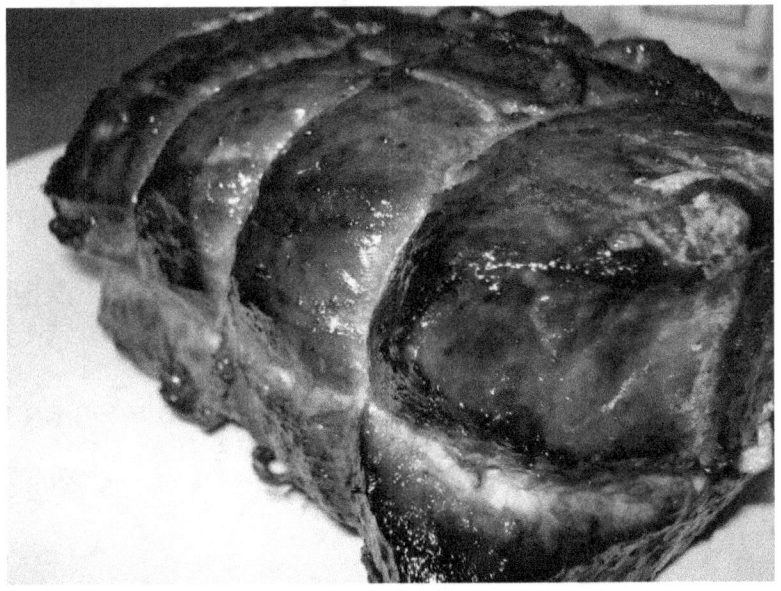

Prep Time: 15 minutes

Cooking Time: 45 minutes

Serving: 6

Ingredients:

- 2 tablespoon steak seasoning rub
- ½ cup balsamic vinegar
- ½ cup olive oil
- 2 pound boneless pork loin roast

Directions:

1. Gently dissolve the steak seasoning in balsamic vinegar
2. Stir them in olive oil and place them in a re-sealable plastic bag

3. Pour the marinade on top of them
4. Squeeze the air out of the bag and seal it up
5. Let it marinade overnight if possible or for at least 2 hours
6. Add the pork into a glass baking dish alongside the marinade
7. Bake it in your pre-heated oven for an hour, making sure to keep basting it from time to time
8. Using a thermometer, check if the internal temperature reaches 145 degrees Fahrenheit
9. Once done, take it out from the oven and let it sit for about 10 minutes
10. Slice and serve!

Nutrition:

- Calories: 299
- Fat: 23.4g
- Carbohydrates: 3.1g
- Protein: 18.3g

Lunch Idea #17 - Marie's Special Easy Peezy Slow Cooker Roast

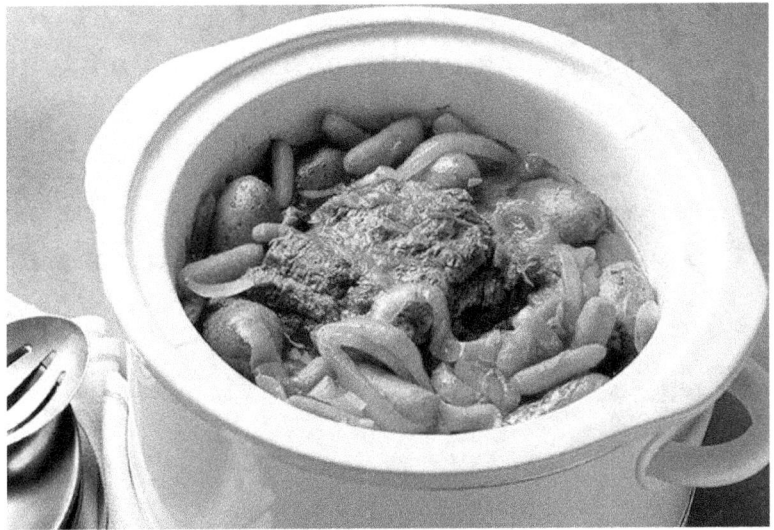

Prep Time: 40 minutes

Cooking Time: 9 hours

Serving: 8

Ingredients:

- 4 pound chuck roast
- Salt as needed
- Pepper as needed
- 1 pack dry onion soup mix
- 1 cup water
- 3 chopped up carrots
- 1 chopped up onion
- 3 peeled and cubed potatoes
- 1 stalk chopped celery

Directions:

1. Season the roast gently with pepper and salt according to your flavor
2. Take a large skillet over high heat and add the seasoned roast
3. Brown both of the roast giving 4 minutes to each side
4. Place the browned roast in your slow cooker and add water, soup mix, carrots, potatoes, onion, and celery
5. Cover up the lid and let it cook on low settings for 8-19 hours
6. Serve hot

Nutrition:

- Calories: 540
- Fat: 30g
- Carbohydrates: 18.2g
- Protein: 45.7g

Lunch Idea #18 - Jalapeno Mixed Turkey Burgers!

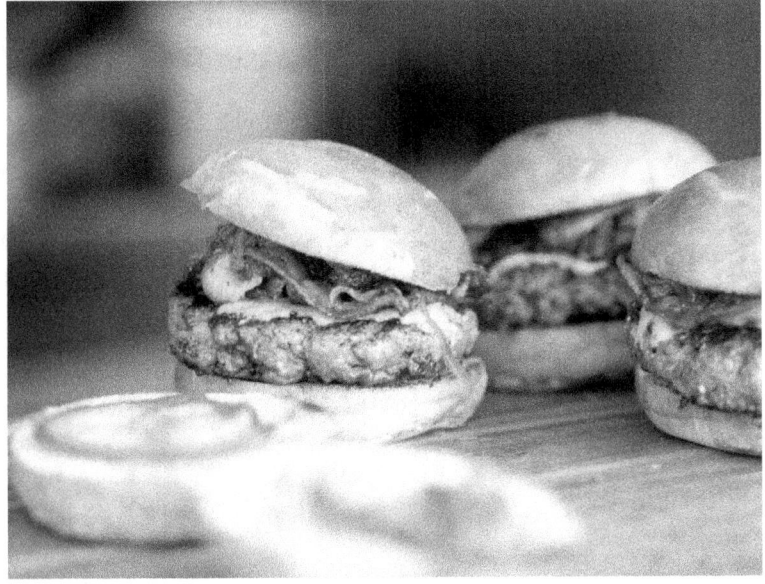

Prep Time: 10 minutes

Cooking Time: 10 minutes

Serving: 4

Ingredients:

- 1 pound ground turkey
- ¾ part minced jalapeno pepper
- 1 medium sized peeled and minced shallot
- Zest just one lime
- 2 teaspoon lime juice
- 2 tablespoon chopped cilantro
- 1 teaspoon paprika
- 1 teaspoon cumin
- ½ teaspoon sea salt

- ½ teaspoon black pepper

Directions:

1. Gently place the turkey, spices, lime and herbs in a fine bowl and use your hand to combine them well
2. Form the mixture into four individual patties
3. Place a pan over medium heat and add olive oil
4. Once the oil is heated up, add the patties and cook them for 5 minutes on each side until they are thoroughly cooked
5. Top it up with some guacamole, poached egg or buns and serve!

Nutrition:

- Calories: 353
- Fat: 16g
- Carbohydrates: 23g
- Protein: 30g

Lunch Idea #19 - Magnificent Slow Cooker Kalua Pig

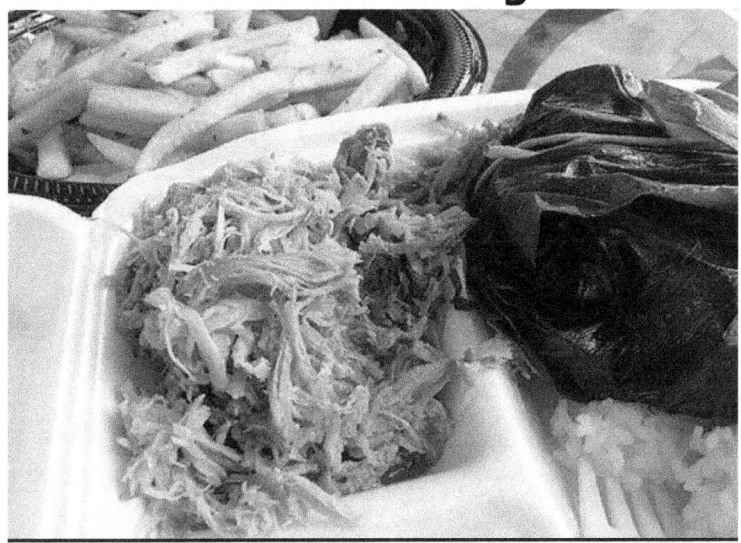

Prep Time: 10 minutes

Cooking Time: 20 hour

Serving: 12

Ingredients:

- 6 pound pork butt roast
- 1 and ½ tablespoon Hawaiian sea salt
- 1 tablespoon liquid smoke flavoring

Directions:

1. Pierce the pork all over with your carving fork
2. Rub salt all over followed by liquid smoke
3. Place the roast in your slow cooker

4. Let it cook on low for 20 hours, making sure to turn it once about halfway through
5. Remove the meat from your cooker
6. Using a fork, shred it apart
7. Add dipping if you need to moisten it and serve hot!

Nutrition:

- Calories: 243
- Fat: 14.7g
- Carbohydrates: 0g
- Protein: 25.9g

Lunch Idea #20 - Indian Chicken Kabobs With Lime And Chili

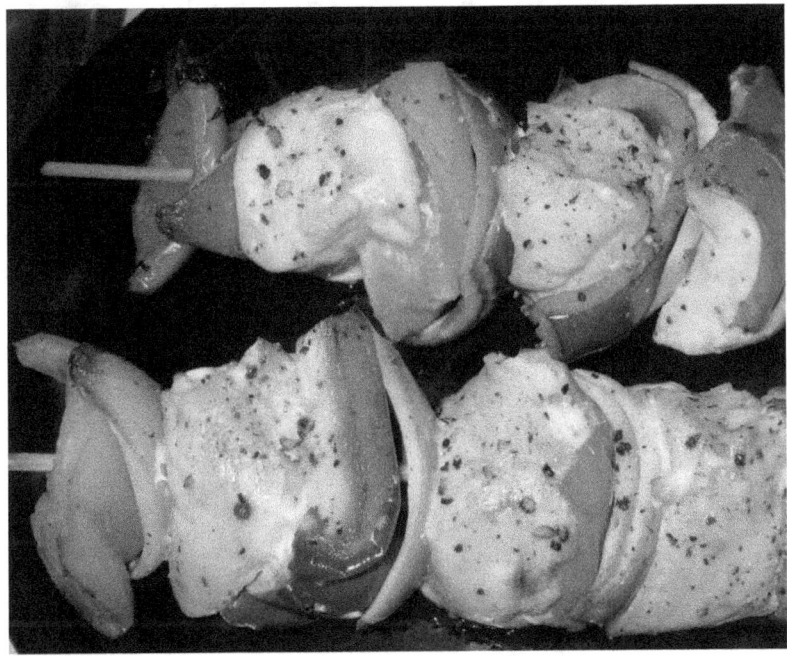

Prep Time: 15 minutes

Cooking Time: 15 minutes

Serving: 4

Ingredients:

- 3 tablespoon olive oil
- 1 and ½ tablespoon red wine vinegar
- 1 juiced lime
- 1 teaspoon chili powder
- ½ teaspoon paprika
- ½ teaspoon onion powder

- ½ teaspoon garlic powder
- Cayenne pepper
- Salt as needed
- Freshly ground pepper as needed
- 1 pound of skinless, boneless halved chicken breast
- Skewers

Directions:

1. Take a small bowl and whisk in the vinegar, olive oil, lime juice
2. Season with some chili powder, onion powder, paprika, garlic powder, salt, cayenne pepper and black pepper
3. Add the chicken in a shallow baking dish with the prepared sauce and stir nicely to coat it up
4. Cover it up and let it marinate for an hour in your fridge
5. Pre-heat your grill for medium-high heat
6. Thread the chicken onto skewers and discard the remaining marinade
7. Lightly oil up the grill grate and grill the skewers for about 10-15 minutes
8. Serve hot!

Nutrition:

- Calories: 227
- Fat: 13g
- Carbohydrates: 3.2g
- Protein: 23.9

Lunch Idea #21 - Highly Spiced Grilled Shrimp

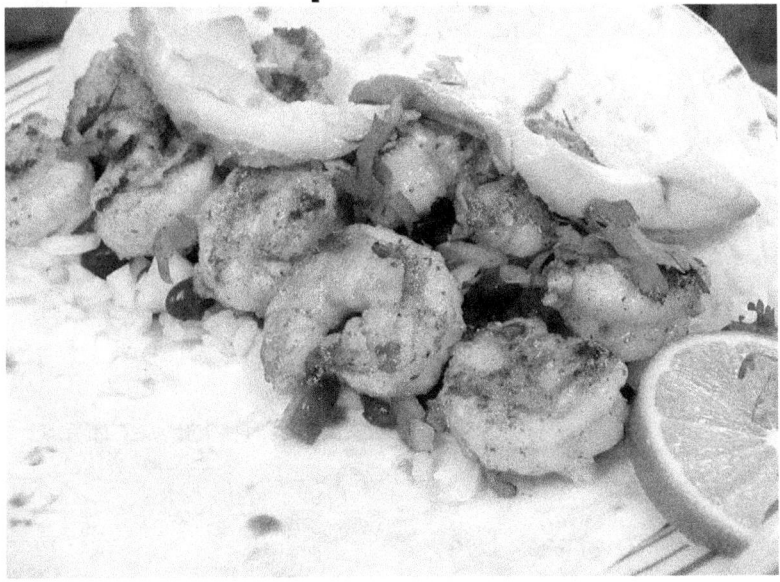

Prep Time: 15 minutes

Cooking Time: 6 minutes

Serving: 6

Ingredients:

- 1 large garlic clove
- 1 tablespoon coarse salt
- ½ tablespoon cayenne pepper
- 1 teaspoon paprika
- 2 tablespoon olive oil
- 2 teaspoon lemon juice
- 2 pound peeled and deveined large shrimp
- 8 wedges lemon

Directions:

1. Pre-heat your grill for medium heat
2. Take a small sized bowl and crush up your garlic with salt
3. Mix in the paprika and Cayenne pepper
4. Stir in olive oil, lemon juice to form a fine paste
5. Take a large sized bowl and toss the shrimp with garlic paste until they are finely coated
6. Lightly grill up your oil grate
7. Cook your shrimp for 2-3 minutes per side
8. Serve with a garnish of lemon wedges

Nutrition:

- Calories: 164
- Fat: 5.9g
- Carbohydrates: 2.7g
- Protein: 25g

Lunch Idea #22 - Zingy Tenderloins

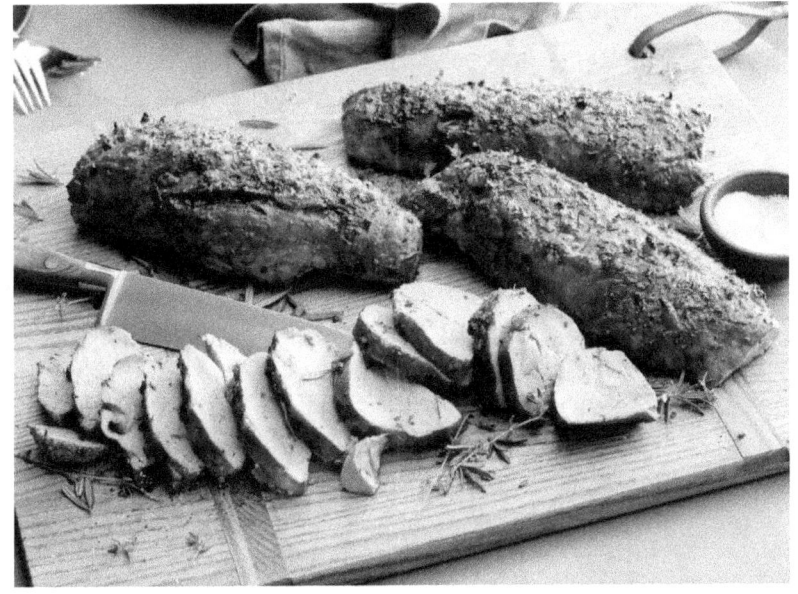

Prep Time: 15 minutes

Cooking Time: 30 minutes

Serving: 6

Ingredients:

- 1 and ½ cup fresh lime juice
- ¾ cup olive oil
- 6 sliced garlic cloves
- 2 teaspoon salt
- 6 tablespoon dried oregano
- 1 pound pork tenderloins

Directions:

1. Take a large re-saleable plastic bag and add lime juice, garlic, olive oil, oregano, and salt
2. Shake the bag until everything is mixed well
3. Taste the marinade for your desired level of tartness
4. Add lemon for more zing or oil for more tart
5. Add the tenderloins to the bag and seal it up
6. Let it marinate in your fridge for 2-5 hours
7. Pre-heat your grill for medium heat
8. Lightly oil up the grate
9. Discard the marinade and place the tenderloins on the grate and grill for 30 minutes to your desired doneness

Nutrition:

- Calories: 404
- Fat: 31g
- Carbohydrates: 9.1g
- Protein: 24g

Lunch Idea #23 - A Delightful Shrimp Scampi

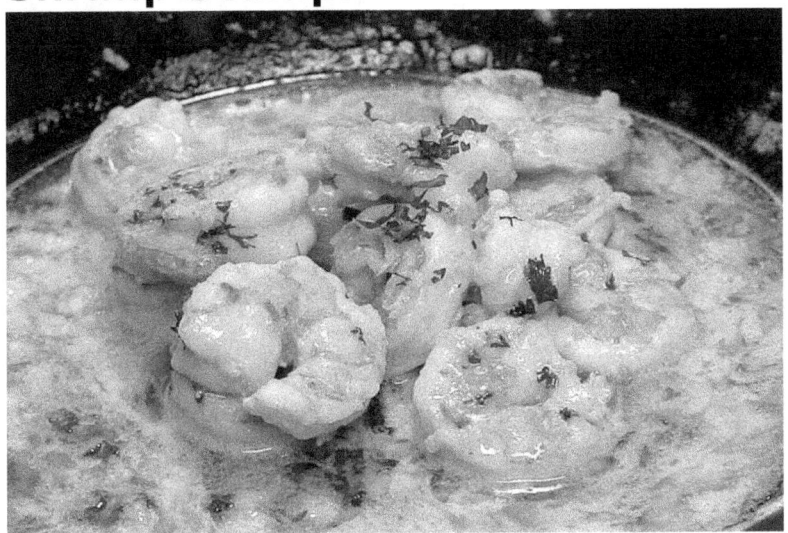

Prep Time: 30 minutes

Cooking Time: 6 minutes

Serving: 173

Ingredients:

- ¼ cup olive oil
- 1/3 cup lemon juice
- 3 tablespoon chopped up fresh parsley
- 1 tablespoon minced garlic
- Ground black pepper
- Crushed red pepper flakes
- 1 and ½ pound peeled and deveined medium shrimp

Directions:

1. Take a large sized bowl and stir in the olive oil, parsley, lemon juice, black pepper and garlic
2. Season the with crushed red pepper
3. Add the shrimp and toss them nicely to coat
4. Marinate them in your fridge for 30 minutes
5. Pre-heat your grill for high heat
6. Thread the shrimps onto skewers making sure to pierce them from tail to head
7. Lightly oil the grate and cook for 2-3 minutes per side
8. Serve hot!

Nutrition:

- Calories: 173
- Fat: 10g
- Carbohydrates: 1.6g
- Protein: 18.7g

Lunch Idea #24 - Rosemary Chicken With Fries

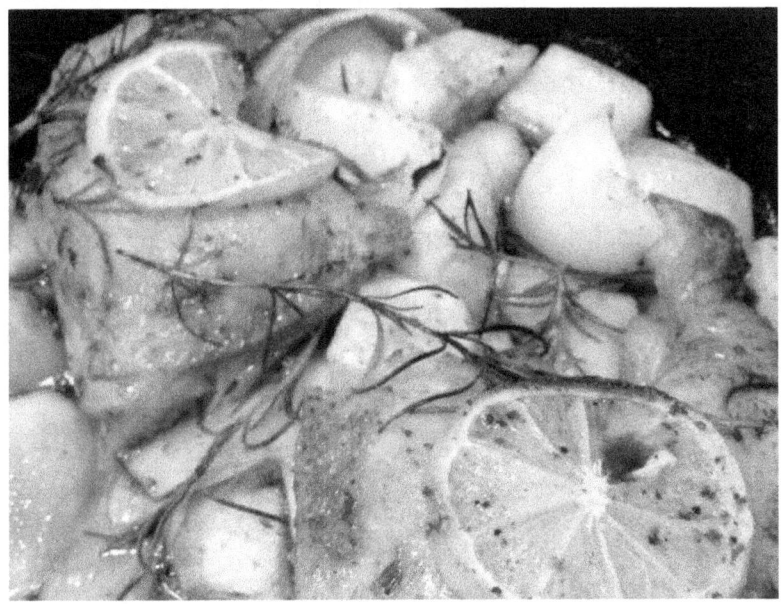

Prep Time: 15 minutes

Cooking Time: 60 minutes

Serving: 6

Ingredients:

- 8 pieces chicken thigh
- 6 small quartered red potatoes
- ½ cup extra virgin olive oil
- 1 tablespoon chopped up fresh rosemary
- 1 and ½ teaspoon chopped up fresh oregano
- 1 and ½ teaspoon garlic powder
- Salt as needed
- Pepper as needed

Directions:

1. Pre-heat your oven to a temperature of 375 degrees Fahrenheit
2. Take a large sized bowl and add the potatoes and chicken
3. Pour olive oil and stir to coat them up
4. Take a large baking dish and scatter the potato pieces and chicken on it
5. Sprinkle some oregano, rosemary, garlic powder, pepper, and salt
6. Bake for about an hour in your oven making sure to Baste it during the final 15 minutes for added crisp

Nutrition:

- Calories: 497
- Fat: 31g
- Carbohydrates: 27g
- Protein: 24.4g

Lunch Idea #25 - Seriously Spicy Mexican Cajun Chicken

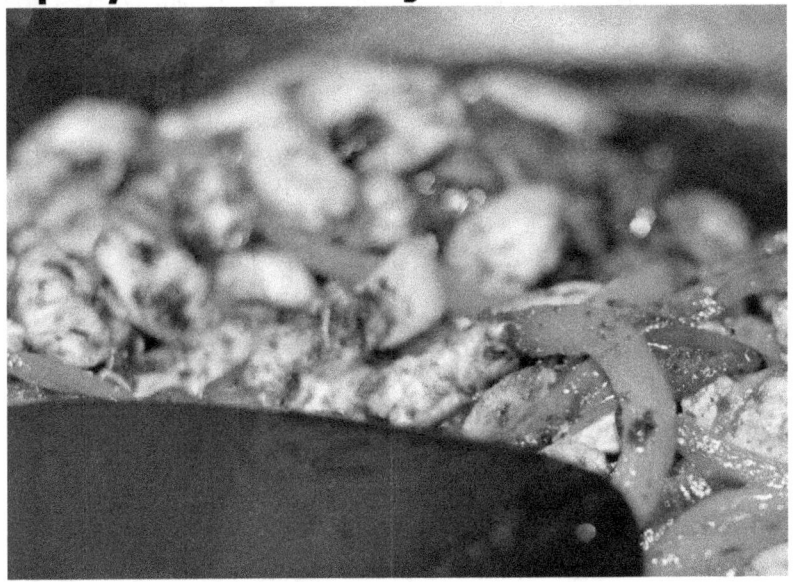

Prep Time: 15 minutes

Cooking Time: 15 minutes

Serving: 6

Ingredients:

- 2 cups vegetable oil
- 2 tablespoon Cajun Seasoning
- 2 tablespoon dried Italian Style Seasoning
- Garlic powder for added flavor
- 2 tablespoon lemon pepper
- 10 boneless and halved chicken breast with their skin removed (pounded to a thickness ½ inch)

Directions:

1. Take a large sized shallow dish
2. Add in the oil, Italian seasoning, Cajun seasoning, lemon pepper and garlic powder
3. Add the chicken to the dish and turn them up once to coat evenly
4. Cover it up and let it refrigerate for ½ an hour
5. Pre-heat your grill for high heat
6. Lightly oil up your grill grate
7. Drain the chicken and toss away the marinade
8. Place the chicken on top of your grill and cook for about 8 minutes per side
9. Serve hot!

Nutrition:

- Calories: 536
- Fat: 47g
- Carbohydrates: 1.8g
- Protein: 26.8g

Lunch Idea #26 - Slow Cooker Mexican Meat

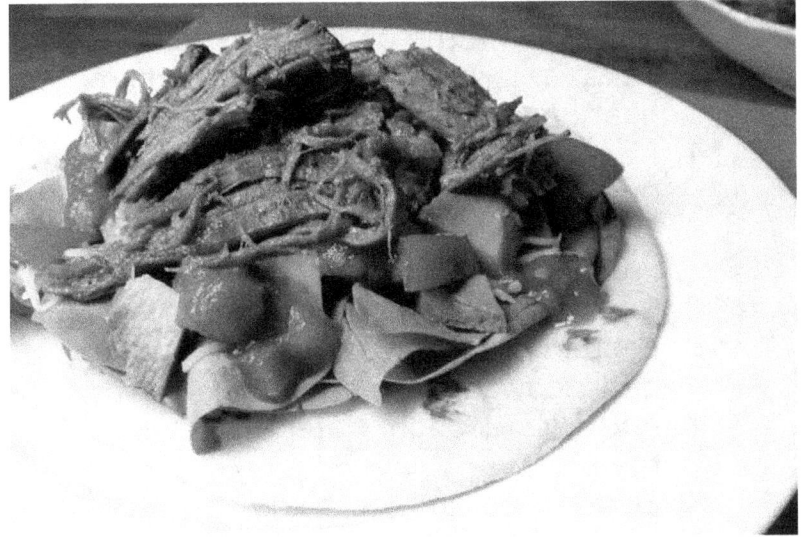

Prep Time: 30 minutes

Cooking Time: 8 hours

Serving: 12

Ingredients:

- 4 pound chuck roast
- 1 teaspoon salt
- 1 teaspoon ground black pepper
- 2 tablespoon olive oil
- 1 large sized chopped onion
- 1 and ¼ cup diced green chili pepper
- 1 teaspoon chili powder
- 1 teaspoon ground cayenne pepper
- 5-ounce bottle hot pepper sauce
- 1 teaspoon garlic powder

Directions:

1. Trim off any of the excess fat from your chuck roast
2. Season with the pepper and salt
3. Take a large skillet over medium-high heat and pour olive oil
4. Place the beef in your skillet and brown on all sides
5. Transfer the roast to your slow cooker and top it up with some chopped onions
6. Season with chili peppers, cayenne pepper, chili powder, hot pepper sauce, garlic powder
7. Add just enough water to cover 1/3 of the roast
8. Cover it up and let it cook on high for 6 hours
9. One the liquid has been reduced to a small amount, reduce the heat to low and cook for another 2-4 hours until the meat is soft
10. Transfer the roast to a bowl and tear it apart using two forks
11. Serve with Rice, Taco's or Burritos!

Nutrition:

- Calories: 260
- Fat: 19g
- Carbohydrates: 3.3g
- Protein: 18g

Lunch Idea #27 - Shivering Cold And Poached Salmon

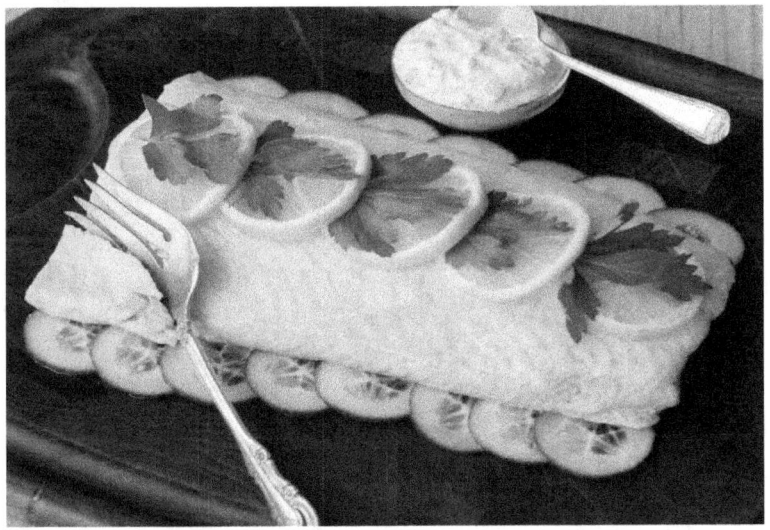

Prep Time: 15 minutes

Cooking Time: 15 minutes

Serving: 4

Ingredients:

- 1 large sized salmon fillet cut up into steaks
- 2 tablespoon olive oil
- 1 chopped up onion
- 3 cloves garlic
- ¼ cup fresh chopped up tarragon
- 1 tablespoon fresh chopped up thyme
- One juice lemon
- 4 cups water
- ½ teaspoon salt
- ¼ teaspoon pepper

Directions:

1. Take a large sized skillet and add olive oil
2. Heat it up
3. Add garlic and onion and cook them until tender
4. Add the lemon, herbs and cook for another minute until the flavors are released
5. Add pepper, salt, and water
6. Bring the mix to a boil and let it simmer for 15 minutes
7. Immerse the salmon into your prepared poaching liquid, making sure that the skin side is facing downwards
8. Cook it for about 12 minutes
9. Once done, remove fish from your liquid and place it on a fine tray
10. Chill it in your fridge for about 3 hours and serve cold!
11. Add some cucumbers if you desire.

Nutrition:

- Calories: 246
- Fat: 14g
- Carbohydrates: 10g
- Protein: 20g

Lunch Idea #28 - Slow Cooked Tangy And Sweet Chicken

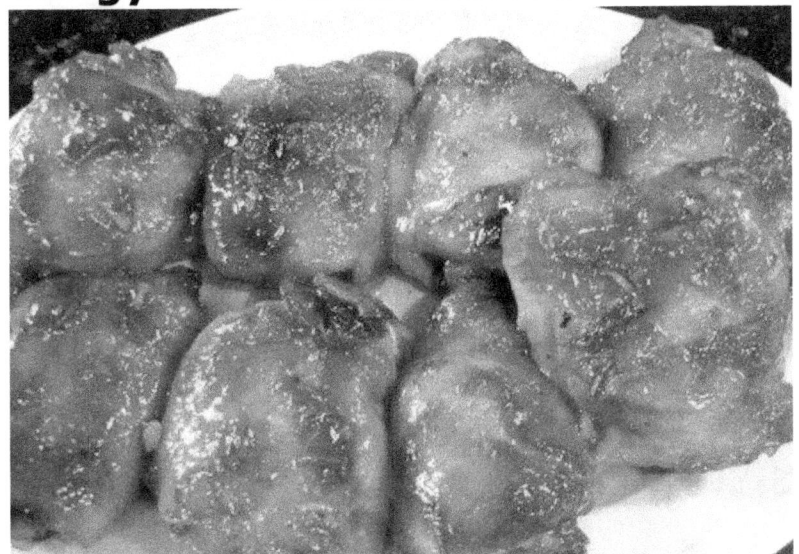

Prep Time: 10 minutes

Cooking Time: 9 hours

Serving: 2

Ingredients:

- 18 ounce BBQ sauce
- 15 ounce pineapple chunks
- 1 chopped up green bell pepper
- 1 chopped up onion
- 2 minced garlic cloves
- 8 boneless and skinless halved chicken breasts

Directions:

1. Take a large sized bowl and mix in the BBQ sauce, pineapple chunks, onion, garlic and green bell pepper
2. Arrange 4 of the breasts in the bottom of your slow cooker
3. Pour half of the BBQ sauce mix
4. Place the rest of the breast
5. Pour the remaining sauce mix on top
6. Cover it up and let it cook for 8-9 hours
7. Serve hot!

Nutrition:

- Calories: 349
- Fat: 2.8g
- Carbohydrates: 56.1g
- Protein: 23g

Lunch Idea #29 - Slow Cooked Bone-In Chicken Thigh

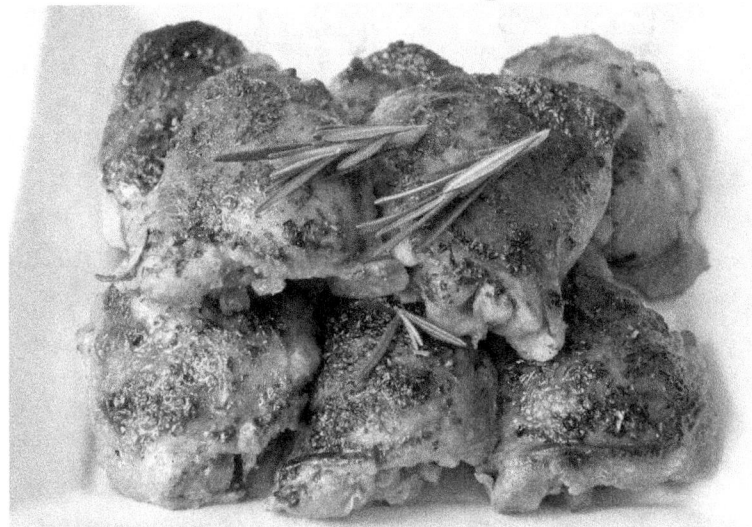

Prep Time: 10 minutes

Cooking Time: 9 hours

Serving: 2

Ingredients:

- Cooking spray
- 8 bone-in chicken thigh skin on
- ¼ teaspoon garlic salt
- ¼ teaspoon onion salt
- ¼ teaspoon dried oregano
- ¼ teaspoon ground thyme
- ¼ teaspoon paprika
- ¼ teaspoon ground black pepper

Directions:

1. Pre-heat your oven to a temperature of 350 degrees Fahrenheit
2. Line up a baking sheet with aluminum foil and spray it with cooking spray
3. Arrange the chicken thigh on your prepared baking sheet
4. Take a small container and combine onion salt, garlic salt, thyme, oregano, paprika and pepper
5. Close up the lid and shake nicely until all of the spices are mixed up
6. Sprinkle the spice mix generously over the thighs
7. Bake the seasoned chicken in your oven for an hour until it is crispy and the bones are no longer pink
8. Use a thermometer to make sure that the internal temperature reads 165 degrees Fahrenheit
9. Serve hot!

Nutrition:

- Calories: 190
- Fat: 11g
- Carbohydrates: 0.2g
- Protein: 19g

Lunch Idea #30 - Magnificent Lobster Tails

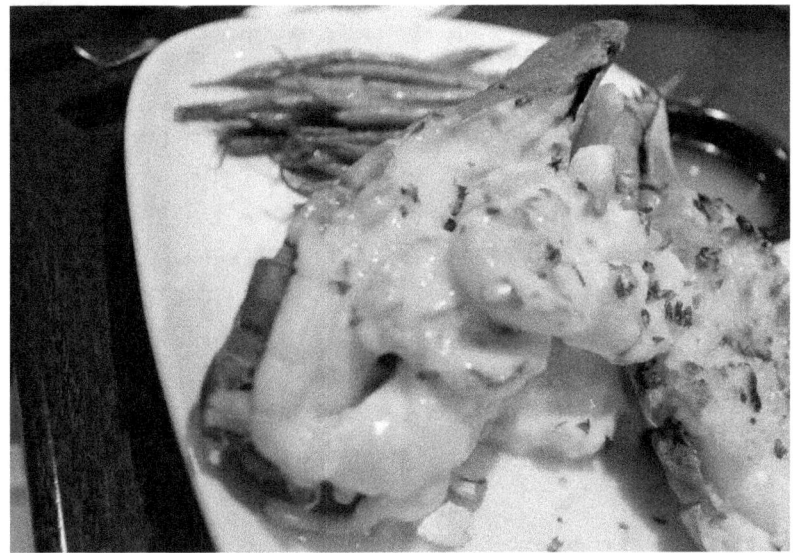

Prep Time: 15 minutes

Cooking Time: 12 minutes

Serving: 2

Ingredients:

- 1 tablespoon lemon juice
- ½ cup olive oil
- 1 teaspoon salt
- 1 teaspoon paprika
- 1/8 teaspoon white pepper
- 1/8 teaspoon garlic powder
- 10 ounce rock lobster tails

Directions:

1. Pre-heat your grill for high-heat

2. Take a small sized bowl and squeeze lemon juice into it
3. Gently whisk in olive oil
4. Then add paprika, salt, garlic powder and white pepper
5. Split the lobster tails lengthwise using a large sized knife and brush the fleshy side of the tail with the prepared marinade
6. Light oil up your grill grate and place the tails with the flesh side facing down
7. Cook for 12 minutes, making sure to turn once and basting it from time to time
8. Discard the excess marinade
9. Serve hot!

Nutrition:

- Calories: 742
- Fat: 60g
- Carbohydrates: 4.3g
- Protein: 44g

Chapter 3: 30 Dinner Ideas

Dinner Idea #1 - Cuban-Style Ropa Vieja

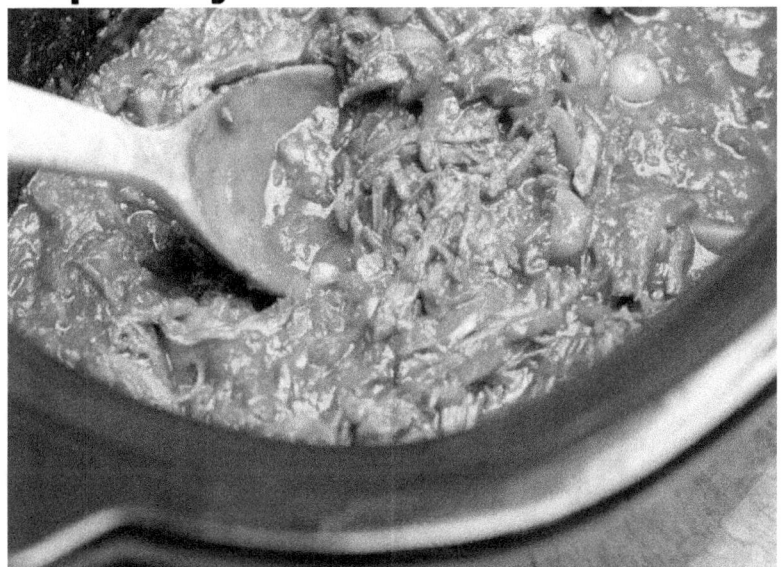

Prep Time: 115minutes

Cooking Time: 4 hours

Serving: 6

Ingredients:

- 1 tablespoon vegetable oil
- 2 pound beef flank steak
- 1 cup beef broth
- 8 ounce tomato sauce
- 1 sliced small onion
- 1 seeded and sliced green bell pepper
- 2 chopped up garlic cloves

- 6 ounce tomato paste
- 1 teaspoon ground cumin
- 1 teaspoon chopped fresh cilantro
- 1 tablespoon of olive oil
- 1 tablespoon of white vinegar

Directions:

1. Take a large sized skillet and pour some vegetable oil
2. Place it over medium-high heat
3. Brown the flanks on either side, cooking each side for 5 minutes
4. Transfer the beef to a slow cooker
5. Pour in the beef broth alongside the tomato sauce
6. Add onion, garlic, bell pepper, cumin, tomato paste, cilantro, vinegar and olive oil
7. Stir it until it is finely blender
8. Cover it up and cook it for 4 hours on high settings
9. Once done, take out the beef and shred it using forks
10. Serve the meat with rice or tortillas

Nutrition:

- Calories: 261
- Fat: 15g
- Carbohydrates: 9.9g
- Protein: 20.5g

Dinner Idea #2 - Summer's Dazzling Shrimp

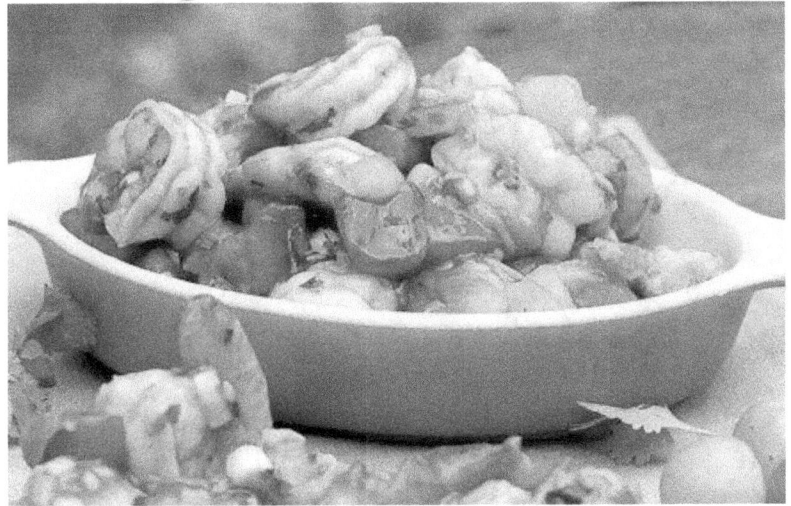

Prep Time: 10 minutes

Cooking Time: 10 minutes

Serving: 6

Ingredients:

- 1/3 cup extra virgin olive oil
- 3 sliced garlic cloves
- 1 teaspoon red pepper flakes
- 2 teaspoon paprika
- 2 pound deveined (shell-on) jumbo shrimp
- ¼ cup lemon juice
- 2 tablespoon chopped fresh basil
- ½ teaspoon salt
- ¼ teaspoon black pepper

Directions:

1. Take a large sized skillet and place it over high heat
2. Pour oil and heat it up
3. Add garlic and stir fry it until translucent
4. Sprinkle some pepper flakes and paprika
5. Add shrimp and toss it gently to coat everything up
6. Pour lemon juice over the shrimp
7. Let the shrimp cook until a bright pink color is shown
8. Once you see that the meat in the center is no longer transparent, cook for another 1-2 minutes
9. Lower down the heat to medium-low and add basil to toss everything finely
10. Season them with some pepper and salt
11. Serve!

Nutrition:

- Calories: 238
- Fat: 13g
- Carbohydrates: 2.2g
- Protein: 25g

Dinner Idea #3 - Mediterranean Style Lemon Chicken

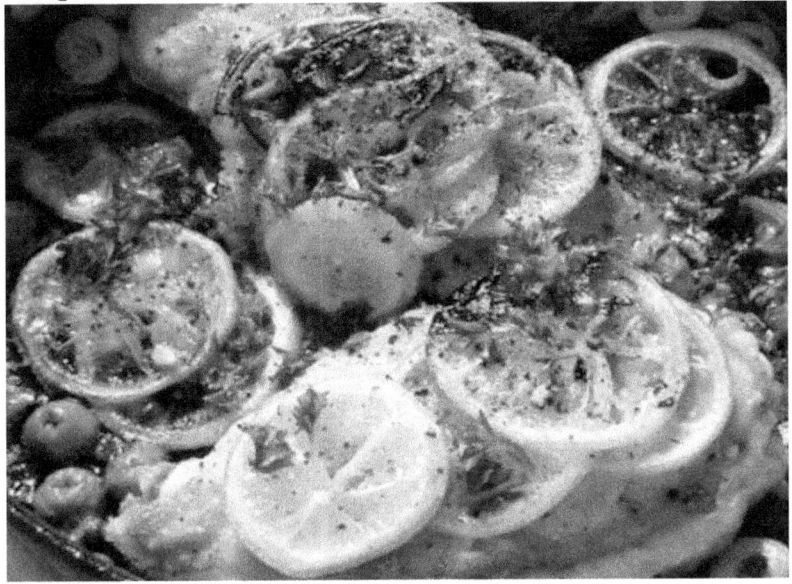

Prep Time: 15 minutes

Cooking Time: 50 minutes

Serving: 6

Ingredients:

- 1 piece lemon
- 2 teaspoon dried oregano
- 3 minced garlic cloves
- 1 tablespoon olive oil
- ¼ teaspoon salt
- ¼ teaspoon ground black pepper
- 5 piece chicken legs

Directions:

1. Pre-heat your oven to a temperature of 425 degrees Fahrenheit
2. Take a large sized 9x13 inch baking dish
3. Grate the peel from ½ of the lemon
4. Take a cup and squeeze the lemon juice
5. Add the peel to your juice with garlic, oregano, pepper and salt
6. Stir the mix until combined
7. Remove the skin from your chicken pieces and toss the away
8. Coat up the chicken with your lemon mix and arrange them finely in your baking dish with the bony side up
9. Cover it up and bake for 20 minutes
10. Turn the chicken and baste with the mix
11. Lower down the heat to 400 degrees Fahrenheit and bake them for 30 minutes uncovered
12. Make sure to keep basting it after every 10 minutes
13. Serve with the pan juices!

Nutrition:

- Calories: 241
- Fat: 11g
- Carbohydrates: 2.8g
- Protein: 30g

Dinner Idea #4 - Indian Styled Aloo Phujia

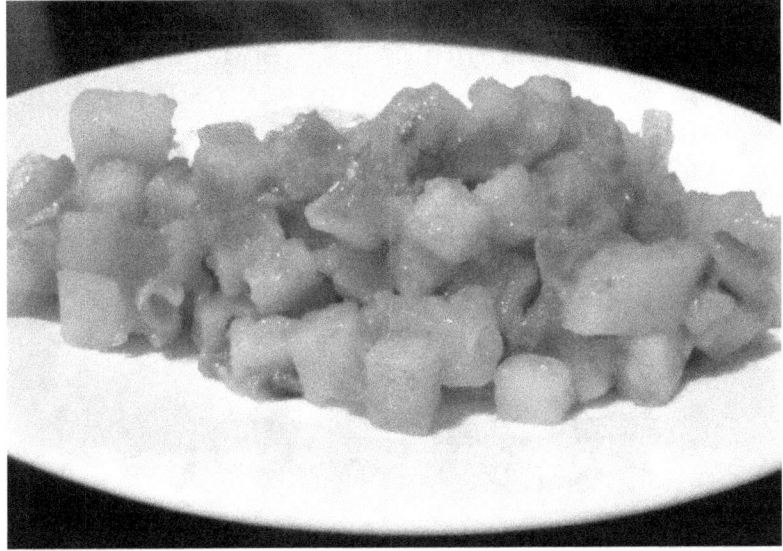

Prep Time: 10 minutes

Cooking Time: 20 minutes

Serving: 4

Ingredients:

- 1 chopped up onion
- ¼ cup vegetable oil
- 1 pound cubed and peeled potatoes
- 1 teaspoon salt
- ½ teaspoon cayenne pepper
- ½ teaspoon cayenne pepper
- ½ teaspoon ground turmeric
- ¼ teaspoon ground cumin
- 2 chopped up tomatoes

Directions:

1. Take a medium sized skillet and place it over medium heat
2. Add the oil and heat it up
3. Add onion to the oil and brown it
4. Stir in the turmeric, cayenne, salt
5. Add the potatoes and keep stirring it for 10 minutes
6. Add tomatoes and over the pan for 10 minutes until the potatoes are tender
7. Serve!

Nutrition:

- Calories: 235
- Fat: 14g
- Carbohydrates: 25g
- Protein: 3.3g

Dinner Idea #5 - Feisty Mojo Marinated Chicken Grill

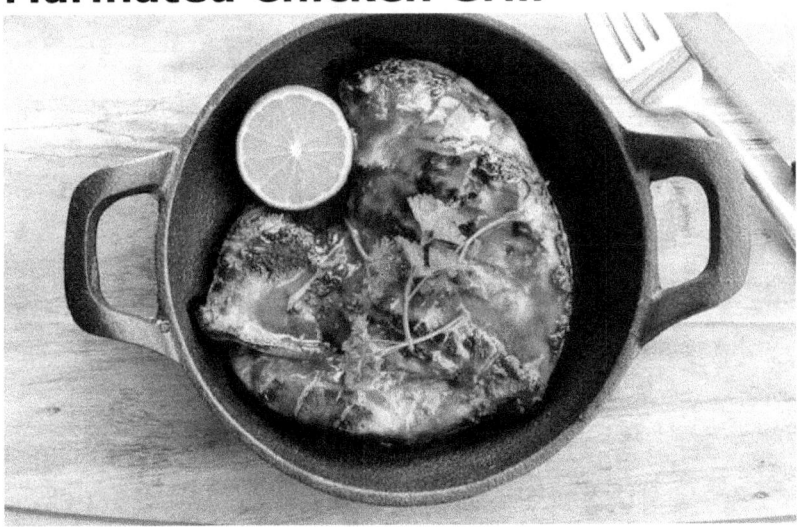

Prep Time: 30 minutes

Cooking Time: 15 minutes

Serving: 4-6

Ingredients:

- 6-8 pieces chicken thigh
- 1 peeled and thickly sliced red onion
- 2 tablespoon olive oil

For the Marinade

- 1 juiced and zested orange
- 3 juiced and zested lime
- 3 minced garlic cloves
- 2 tablespoon of olive oil
- ½ a cup of chicken stock
- 1 tablespoon of ground cumin

- 1 teaspoon of salt
- ¼ teaspoon of ground pepper

Directions:

1. Take a resealable bag and add all of the ingredients listed under marinade and combine them nicely
2. Keep just a quarter of the mix aside for later use
3. Add the chicken pieces to the re-sealable bag and let it marinate for at least 20 minutes
4. Rub olive oil all over the red onion slices and keep them on a platter
5. Heat up the grill to a high setting and place the onions and marinated chicken on top of the grill
6. Lower down the heat to medium-high
7. Cook it for 6 minutes on each side, making sure to keep basting it using the previously reserved marinade
8. Take an internal thermometer and check the temperature of the chicken
9. Once it reaches 165 degrees, it is done!
10. Serve!

Nutrition:

- Calories: 225
- Fat: 13g
- Carbohydrates: 13g
- Protein: 24g

Dinner Idea #6 - Stir Fried Cabbage With Garlic, Onion, and Bacon

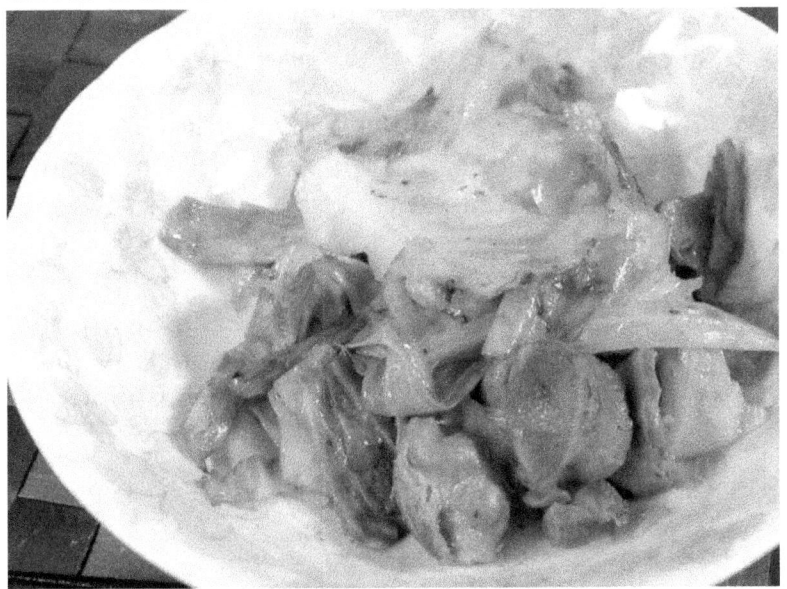

Prep Time: 15 minutes

Cooking Time: 60 minutes

Serving: 6

Ingredients:

- 6 large sized chopped bacon
- 1 diced large onion
- 2 minced garlic cloves
- 1 large cabbage head sliced and cored
- 1 tablespoon salt
- 1 teaspoon ground black pepper
- ½ teaspoon onion powder
- ½ teaspoon garlic powder

- 1/8 teaspoon paprika

Directions:

1. Take a large sized stock pot and place it over medium-high heat
2. Add bacon and cook for 10 minutes until crispy
3. Add onions followed by garlic and cook for another 10 minutes until the onions are caramelized
4. Stir in the cabbage and keep cooking for another 10 minutes
5. Season with some pepper, salt, garlic powder, onion powder and paprika
6. Lower down the heat and simmer for 30 minutes more
7. Serve!

Nutrition:

- Calories: 194
- Fat: 12g
- Carbohydrates: 15g
- Protein: 6g

Dinner Idea #7 - Sugary Snapped Peas

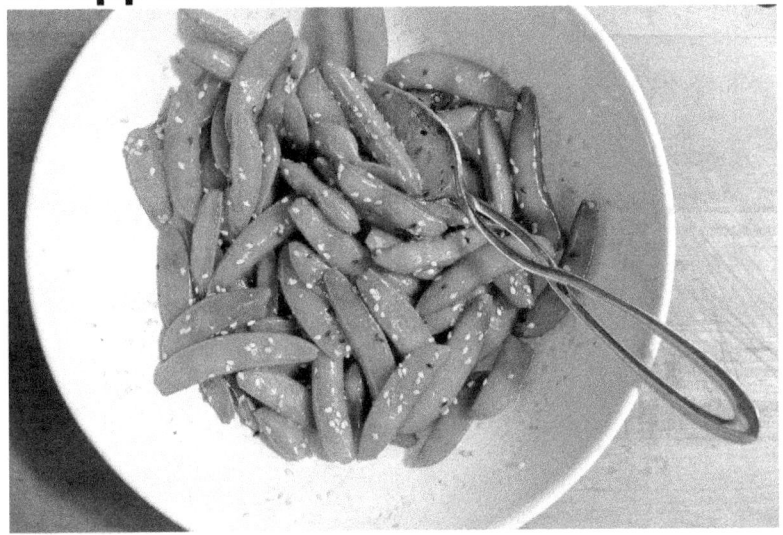

Prep Time: 10 minutes

Cooking Time: 8 minutes

Serving: 6

Ingredients:

- ½ pound sugar snap peas
- 1 tablespoon olive oil
- 1 tablespoon chopped shallots
- 1 teaspoon chopped up fresh thyme
- Kosher salt as needed

Directions:

1. Pre-heat your oven to a temperature of 450 degrees Fahrenheit
2. Take a baking sheet and add the sugar snap peas, forming a fine single layer

3. Brush them up with some olive oil
4. Sprinkle with thyme, shallots and kosher salt
5. Bake in your pre-heated oven for 6-8 minutes
6. Serve when soft yet firm

Nutrition:

- Calories: 59
- Fat: 3.4g
- Carbohydrates: 5.3g
- Protein: 1.4g

Dinner Idea #8 - The Widely (Loved) Pineapple Pork Roast

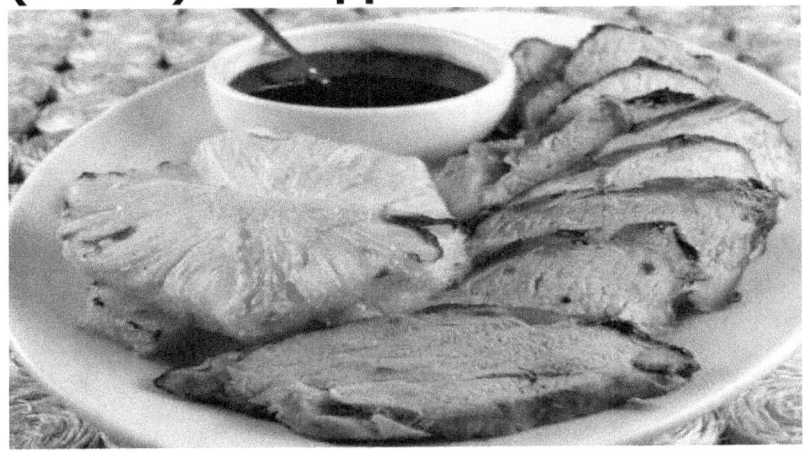

Prep Time: 15 minutes

Cooking Time: 7 hours

Serving: 6

Ingredients:

- 3 pound boneless pork roast
- 2 teaspoon seasoned salt
- 1 teaspoon ground black pepper
- 20-ounce pineapple chunks
- 1 and ½ cup chopped up dried cranberries

Directions:

1. Rub and season your pork with pepper and salt on all sides
2. Place the pork in your slow cookers
3. Pour in the pineapple chunks alongside

4. Cover it up and let it cook for 7 hours on low settings
5. Serve!

Nutrition:

- Calories: 339
- Fat: 8.9g
- Carbohydrates: 40g
- Protein: 26g

Dinner Idea #9 - A Watermelon Salsa Of Fire and Ice

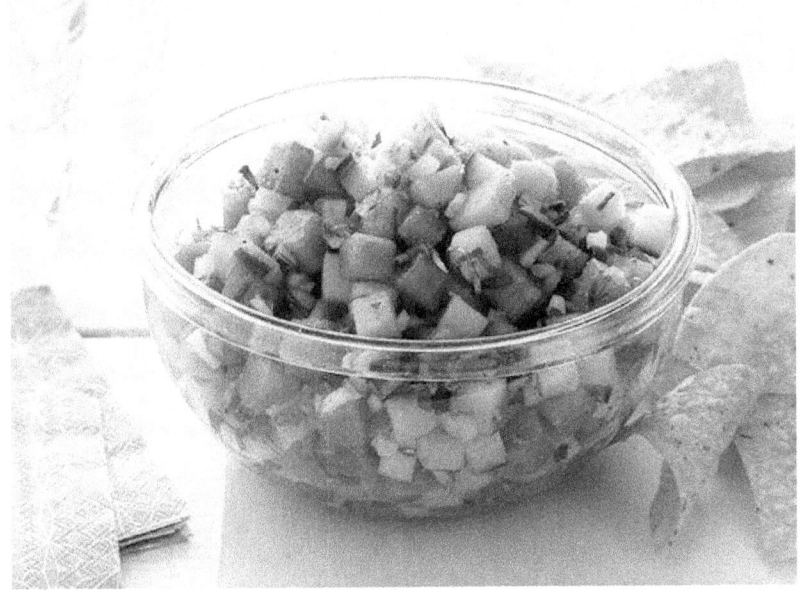

Prep Time: 15 minutes

Cooking Time: 15 minutes

Serving: 6

Ingredients:

- 3 cups chopped up watermelon
- ½ cup chopped up green bell pepper
- 2 tablespoon lime juice
- 2 tablespoon chopped up fresh cilantro
- 1 tablespoon chopped up jalapeno pepper
- ½ teaspoon garlic salt

Directions:

1. Take a large sized bowl and add watermelon, lime juice, green bell pepper, green onions, cilantro, jalapeno, and garlic salt
2. Mix them well
3. Serve Chilled!

Nutrition:

- Calories: 5
- Fat: 0g
- Carbohydrates: 1.3g
- Protein: 0.1g

Dinner Idea #10 - Chicken Soup Base From Scratch

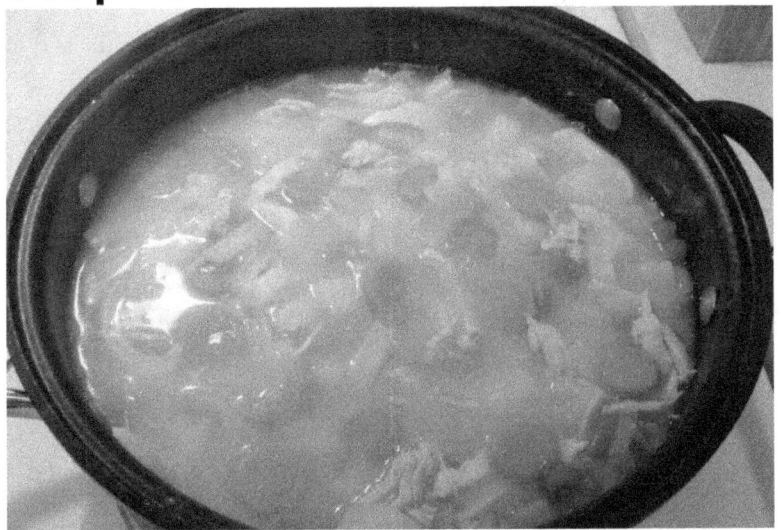

Prep Time: 10 minutes

Cooking Time: 40 minutes

Serving: 8

Ingredients:

- 2 quarts chicken broth
- 1 quart of water
- 1 store-bought chicken roast
- 3 tablespoon vegetable oil
- 2 large sized onion cut up into medium dice
- 2 large sized peeled carrots cut up into rounds
- 2 large celery stalks sliced into ¼ thick slices
- 1 teaspoon dried thyme leaves

Directions:

1. Take a soup kettle and place it over medium-high heat
2. Add the water and broth bring it to a simmer
3. In the meantime, separate the chicken meat from the skin and the bones of your roast
4. Add the skin and bones into the simmering pot
5. Lower down the heat to low and cover it up
6. Simmer for 20-30 minutes to allow the bone to release their flavor
7. Strain the broth through a colander into a large sized container
8. Keep the broth for later use and discard the bones and skin
9. Return it to a burner and set the burner to medium-high heat
10. Add oil, carrots, onion and celery to the kettle
11. Sauté them for about 10 minutes until they are soft
12. Add chicken meat, thyme and broth
13. Bring the mix to simmer
14. Serve hot!

Nutrition:

- Calories: 338
- Fat: 21g
- Carbohydrates: 5.8g
- Protein: 29g

Dinner Idea #11 - Fish Stew From The Depths Of Brazil

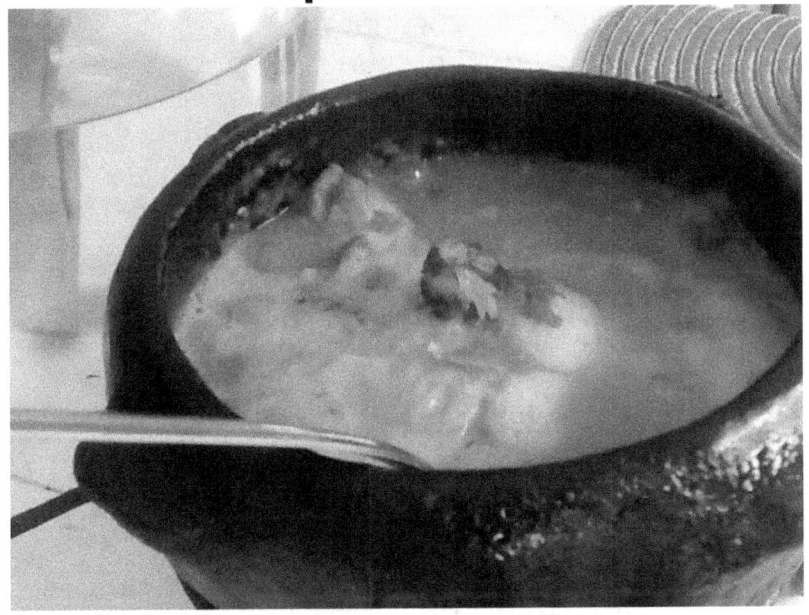

Prep Time: 20 minutes

Cooking Time: 25 minutes

Serving: 8

Ingredients:

- 3 tablespoon lime juice
- 1 tablespoon ground cumin
- 1 tablespoon paprika
- 2 teaspoon minced garlic
- 1 teaspoon salt
- 1 teaspoon black pepper
- 1 and ½ pound tilapia fillet cut up into chunks
- 2 tablespoon olive oil

- 2 chopped onions
- 4 sliced large bell peppers
- 16 ounce diced and drained tomatoes
- 16 ounce of coconut milk
- 1 bunch of chopped of cilantro

Directions:

1. Take a bowl and add in the cumin, lime juice, garlic, paprika, pepper, and salt
2. Add tilapia and stir it nicely to toss it evenly coat
3. Cover it up and let it refrigerate for 20 minutes or for 24 hours
4. Take a large sized pot and place it over medium-high heat
5. Pour olive oil and heat it up
6. Add onions to the oil and cook for 2 minutes
7. Lower down the heat to medium
8. Add tilapia, bell peppers, diced up tomatoes to the pot in following layers
9. Cover it up and simmer for 15 minutes, making sure to keep stirring
10. Stir in the cilantro then and keep cooking for 5-10 minutes more
11. Serve hot!

Nutrition:

- Calories: 359
- Fat: 21g
- Carbohydrates: 15g
- Protein: 27g

Dinner Idea #12 - The Original Hungarian Goulash

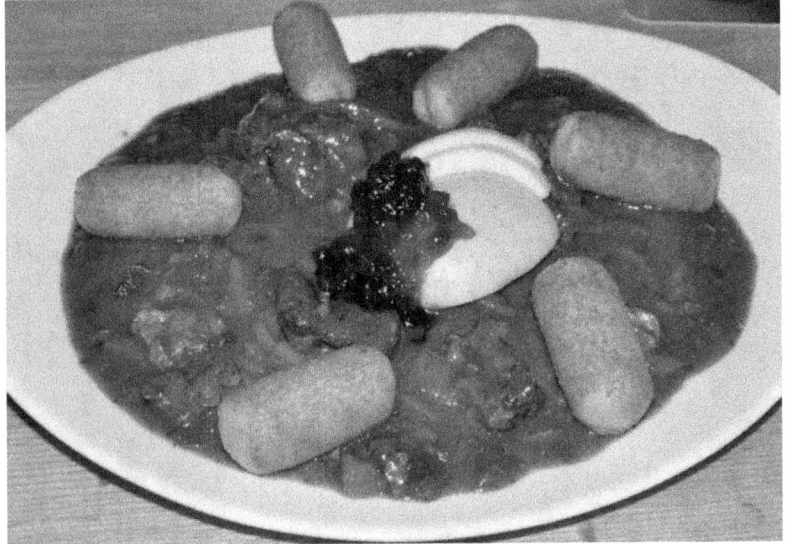

Prep Time: 15 minutes

Cooking Time: 120 minutes

Serving: 8

Ingredients:

- 3 tablespoon lime juice
- 1 tablespoon ground cumin
- 1 tablespoon paprika
- 2 teaspoon minced garlic
- 1 teaspoon salt
- 1 teaspoon black pepper
- 1 and ½ pound tilapia fillet cut up into chunks
- 2 tablespoon olive oil
- 2 chopped onions

- 4 sliced large bell peppers
- 16 ounce diced and drained tomatoes
- 16 ounce coconut milk
- 1 bunch chopped of cilantro

Directions:

1. Take a large sized pot and place it over medium heat
2. Pour oil and heat it up
3. Add onions and cook it until they are soft
4. Remove the onions once cooked and put them on the side
5. Take a medium sized bowl and add paprika, pepper, 2 teaspoons of salt and the beef cubes
6. Toss them to mix the cubes in the spice mix nicely
7. Cook them in the pot until they are browned on all sides
8. Return the onions to the pot then and pour tomato paste, garlic, water and the rest of the remaining 1 teaspoon of salt
9. Lower down the heat and cover it up
10. Let it simmer for around 2 hours until the meat is soft
11. Serve hot!

Nutrition:

- Calories: 549
- Fat: 42g
- Carbohydrates: 9.4g
- Protein: 32g

Dinner Idea #13 - Happy Mother's Turkey Sausage

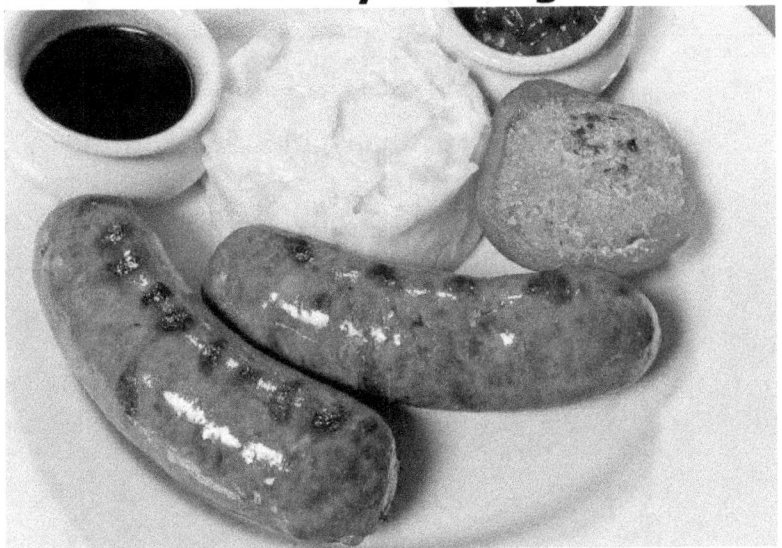

Prep Time: 5 minutes

Cooking Time: 15 minutes

Serving: 8

Ingredients:

- 2 pounds ground turkey
- ¾ teaspoon ground ginger
- 1 and ½ teaspoon salt
- 1 teaspoon dried sage
- ¼ teaspoon cayenne pepper
- 1 and ½ teaspoon ground black pepper

Directions:

1. Take a large sized bowl and mix in the ginger, ground turkey, salt, cayenne

pepper, sage and black pepper until they are blended finely
2. Take a skillet and place it over medium-high heat
3. Coat it up with some non-stick cooking spray
4. Form the previously blender turkey mix into patties
5. Fry them for 15 minutes until they are browned on either side

Nutrition:

- Calories: 169
- Fat: 8.6g
- Carbohydrates: 0.5g
- Protein: 22.5g

Dinner Idea #14 - Unique Margarita Grilled Shrimp

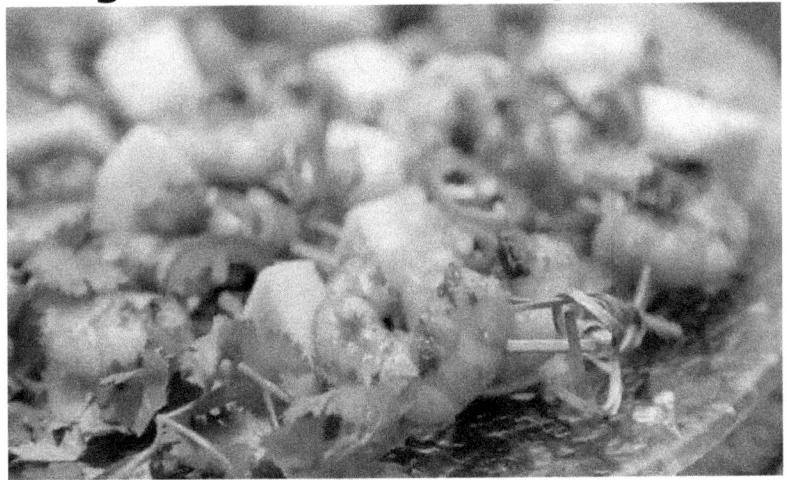

Prep Time: 15 minutes

Cooking Time: 5 minutes

Serving: 4

Ingredients:

- 1 pound peeled and deveined shrimp
- 3 tablespoon olive oil
- 3 tablespoon chopped up fresh cilantro
- 2 tablespoon fresh lime juice
- 2 minced garlic cloves
- 2 teaspoon tequila
- ¼ teaspoon cayenne pepper
- ¼ teaspoon salt
- 4 bamboo skewers soaked up in water for 20 minutes

Directions:

1. Take a bowl and add shrimp, cilantro, olive oil, garlic, lime juice, cayenne, and tequila
2. Cover up the bowl with a plastic wrap and let it refrigerate for 30 minutes
3. Pre-heat your outdoor grill for high-heat and lightly grate up your oil
4. Remove the marinated shrimp from the bowl and thread them onto your skewers
5. Discard the marinade
6. Cook on your pre-heated grill for 2-3 minutes per side, until the shrimp turns pink

Nutrition:

- Calories: 188
- Fat: 11g
- Carbohydrates: 1.3g
- Protein: 18g

Dinner Idea #15 - The Genuine African Chicken Curry

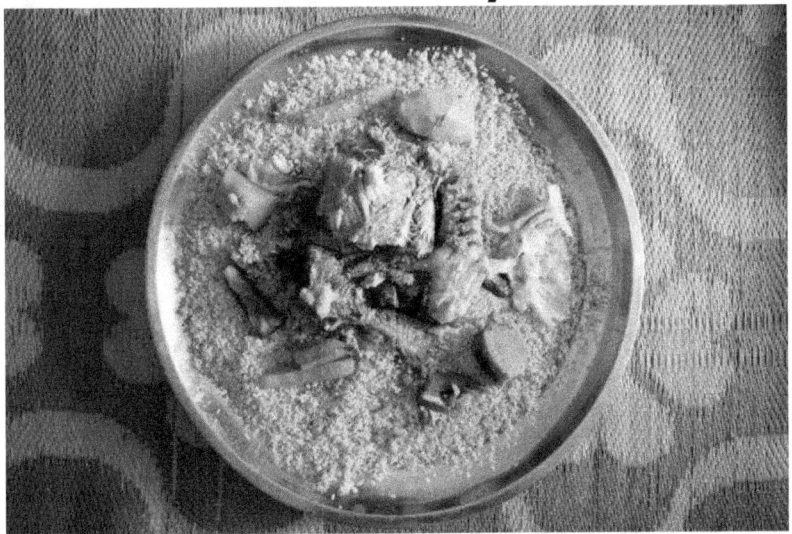

Prep Time: 20 minutes

Cooking Time: 40 minutes

Serving: 4

Ingredients:

- 1 tablespoon olive oil
- 1 chopped up onion
- 2 cloves peeled and chopped garlic cloves
- 1 bay leaf
- 14 ounce whole peeled and drained tomatoes
- 2 teaspoon curry powder
- 1/8 teaspoon salt
- 1 whole chicken with its bones and skin removed (cut up into small pieces)

- 14 ounce unsweetened coconut milk
- 1 juice lemon

Directions:

1. Take a large sized heavy skillet and place t over medium heat
2. Pour olive oil and heat it up
3. Stir in garlic, onion and bay leaf
4. Sauté them until lightly browned
5. Mix up the tomatoes, salt and curry powder to the skillet
6. Keep cooking for another 5 minutes
7. Mix the chicken and cook for another 20 minutes until the meat it no longer pink
8. Lower down the heat to low
9. Keep stirring is constantly and blend the coconut milk for about 10 minutes
10. Mix in the lemon juice and serve!

Nutrition:

- Calories: 600
- Fat: 33g
- Carbohydrates: 13g
- Protein: 64g

Dinner Idea #16 - A Gentle Salad of Avocado and Cucumber

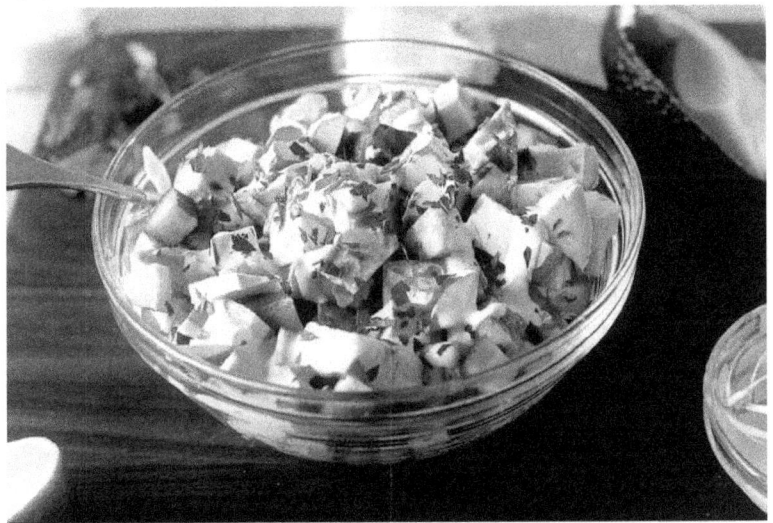

Prep Time: 15 minutes

Cooking Time: 0 minute

Serving: 4

Ingredients:

- 2 cubed medium cucumbers
- 2 cubed avocados
- 4 tablespoon of chopped up fresh cilantro
- 1 minced garlic clove
- 2 tablespoon minced green onions
- ¼ teaspoon salt
- Black pepper as needed
- Black pepper as needed
- ¼ large lemon
- 1 lime

Directions:

1. Take a large sized bowl and combine the avocados, cucumbers, and cilantro
2. Stir in the onions, garlic, pepper and salt
3. Squeeze in lemon and lime all over and toss gently to mix them up
4. Let it refrigerate for 30 minutes and serve chilled!

Nutrition:

- Calories: 186
- Fat: 14g
- Carbohydrates: 15g
- Protein: 3.1g

Dinner Idea #17 - Very Spicy (Original) Thai Soup

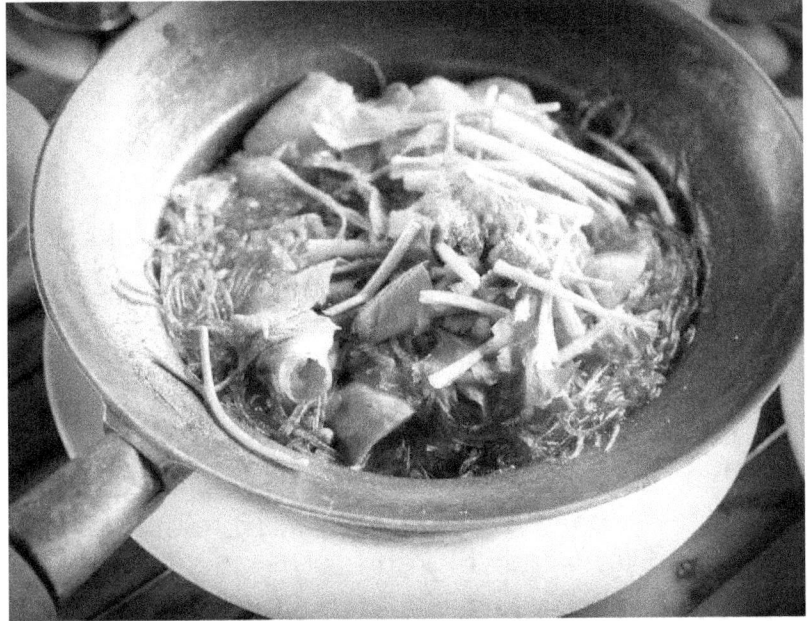

Prep Time: 15 minutes

Cooking Time: 60 minutes

Serving: 6

Ingredients:

- 3 thinly sliced lemon grass stalks
- 4 chopped garlic cloves
- 4 inch chopped ginger root
- 4 cups chicken broth
- 1 tablespoon vegetable oil
- 2 and ½ pound of boneless and skinless chicken thigh (Cut up into small chunks)
- 12 ounce quartered white mushrooms
- 2 teaspoon red curry paste

- 3 tablespoon fish sauce
- 1 juice lime
- 14 ounce of coconut milk
- 1 sliced red onion
- ½ bunch of roughly chopped cilantro
- 1 lime cut up into wedges
- 1 fresh jalapeno pepper sliced up into rings

Directions:

1. Take a stock pot and place it over medium-high heat
2. Stir in lemon grass, ginger, and garlic
3. Stir in the chicken broth and bring the mix to a boil
4. Lower down the heat once boiling point is reached and simmer for 30 minutes
5. Strain the chicken broth and set it aside
6. Discard the garlic, lemon grass, and ginger
7. Take a large soup pot and place it over medium heat
8. Heat some vegetable oil
9. Stir in the chicken and stir-fry for 5 minutes
10. Stir in the mushrooms and cook for another 5 minutes
11. Stir in the red curry paste, lime juice, and fish sauce until they are finely combined
12. Stir in the coconut milk and chicken broth to the mix
13. Return the mix to a simmer and cook on low for about 15 -20 minutes

14.   Skin of the excess oil from top

15.   Stir in the red onions into the chicken mix and cook for 5 minutes until the onions are tender

16.   Serve!

Nutrition:

- Calories: 596
- Fat: 44g
- Carbohydrates: 14g
- Protein: 41g

Dinner Idea #18 - The Best Chicken Stew From Italy

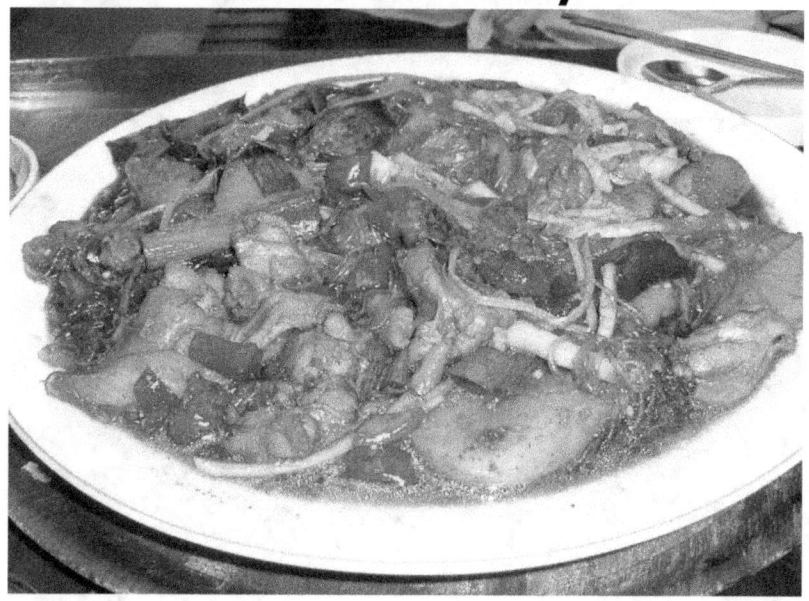

Prep Time: 5 minutes

Cooking Time: 25 minutes

Serving: 4

Ingredients:

- 2 tablespoon olive oil
- 1 pound chicken breast cut up into small pieces
- 1 chopped up large onion
- 3 carrots cut up into bite sized portions
- 2 garlic cloves
- 1 piece Portobello mushroom (stem removed and cut up into bite-sized portions)

- 1/3 cup chopped up parsley
- 3 tablespoon tomato paste
- 14.5 ounce chopped tomatoes
- ½ cup chicken broth
- 2 teaspoon of cinnamon
- Crumbled feat
- Whole wheat couscous

Directions:

1. Take a soup pot and heat up your olive oil
2. Add the chicken and Sauté them until slightly brown
3. Remove the chicken from your pan alongside 1 tablespoon of oil
4. Add carrots onion, pepper and salt
5. Sauté the vegetables until they are tender
6. Add garlic and Sauté for another minute
7. Add parsley and mushrooms and simmer for another 5 minutes
8. Add the previously browned chicken to the pot now
9. Add canned chopped tomatoes, tomato paste, chicken broth and beef broth
10. Stir the mix well and simmer for about 20 minutes
11. Dust them with some cinnamon
12. Serve with some sprinkled Feta or Couscous

Nutrition:

- Calories: 881
- Fat: 10g

- Carbohydrates: 128g
- Protein: 71g

Dinner Idea #19 - The Native American Date and Bacon Wrap

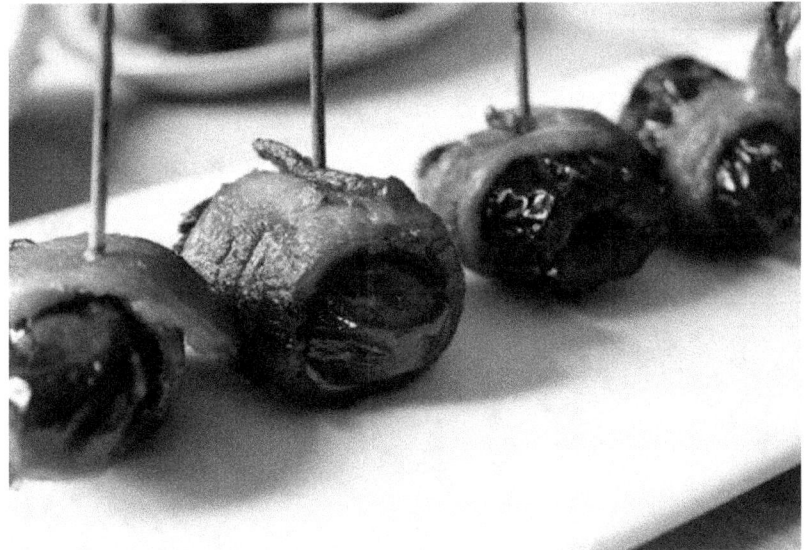

Prep Time: 30 minutes

Cooking Time: 5 minutes

Serving: 6

Ingredients:

- 8 ounce pitted dates
- 4 ounce almonds
- 1 pound sliced bacon

Directions:

1. Pre-heat your broiler and prepare it first
2. Slit the dates and place one almond inside each of the dates

3. Wrap the dates up with bacon and pierce a toothpick through it to ensure that they are tightly held together
4. Broil for about 10 minutes until the bacon is finely crisp and brown
5. Serve!

Nutrition:

- Calories: 560
- Fat: 43g
- Carbohydrates: 32g
- Protein: 13g

Dinner Idea #20 - Sweet Minestrone Soup

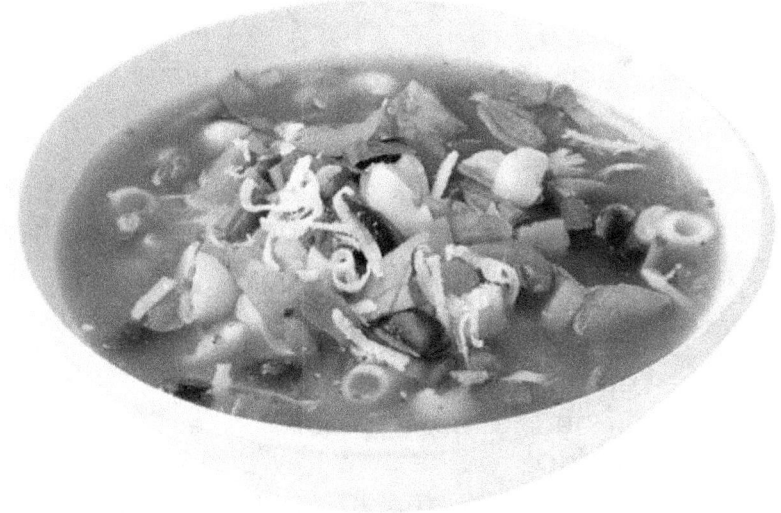

Prep Time: 30 minutes

Cooking Time: 5 minutes

Serving: 6

Ingredients:

- 1 tablespoon vegetable oil
- 1 chopped up large onion
- 2 chopped up large celery stalks
- 2 and ½ teaspoon Italian seasoning
- Salt as needed
- Pepper as needed
- 28 ounce Italian Style Diced Tomatoes
- 5 cups vegetable broth
- 2 large peeled and diced sweet potatoes

- 2 large thinly sliced carrots
- 6 ounce green beans cut up into 1-inch pieces
- 5 minced garlic cloves

Directions:

1. Take a soup pot and place it over medium-high heat
2. Heat up some oil
3. Add the onions, Italian seasoning, pepper, salt, and onion and Sauté them for 5 minutes until soft
4. Stir in the tomatoes alongside its juice, sweet potatoes, broth, carrots, garlic and green beans
5. Bring the mix to a boil
6. Reduce the heat to low and simmer it for 30 minutes, making sure to keep stirring it from time to time
7. Once the vegetables are soft, serve hot!

Nutrition:

- Calories: 201
- Fat: 2.7g
- Carbohydrates: 39g
- Protein: 4.5g

Dinner Idea #21 - The Original Tom Ka Gai

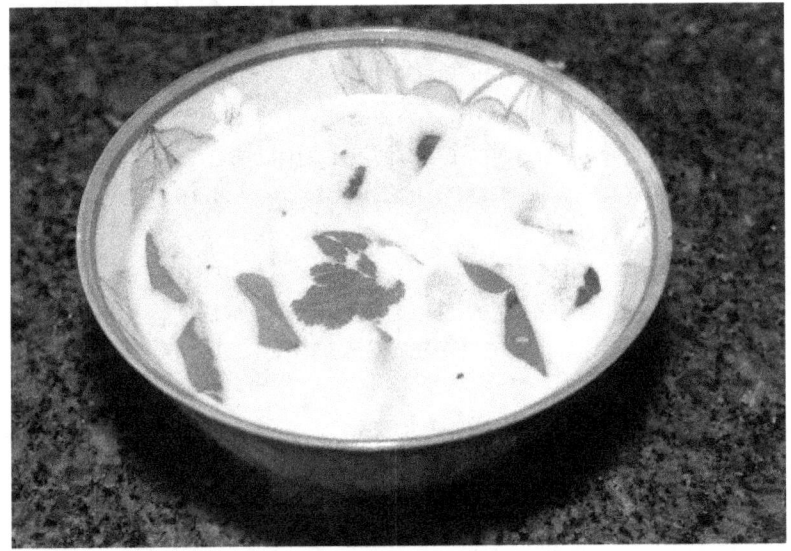

Prep Time: 30 minutes

Cooking Time: 5 minutes

Serving: 6

Ingredients:

- ¾ pound skinless, boneless chicken meat
- 3 tablespoon vegetable oil
- 14 ounce coconut milk
- 2 cups water
- 2 tablespoon minced fresh ginger root
- 4 tablespoon fish sauce
- ¼ cup lime juice
- ¼ teaspoon cayenne pepper
- ½ teaspoon turmeric
- 2 tablespoon thinly sliced green onion
- 1 tablespoon freshly chopped cilantro

Directions:

1. Cut up the chicken into thin strips and Sauté them in oil for about 2-3 minutes
2. Take a pot and add the coconut milk and water
3. Bring the mix to a boil
4. Lower down the heat and add fish sauce, ginger, lime juice, turmeric and cayenne powder
5. Simmer the chicken for 15 minutes
6. Sprinkle with some fresh cilantro, scallions and serve while hot!

Nutrition:

- Calories: 433
- Fat: 41g
- Carbohydrates: 5.5g
- Protein: 14.8g

Dinner Idea #22 - Delightful Whole Foods Omelet Cupcakes

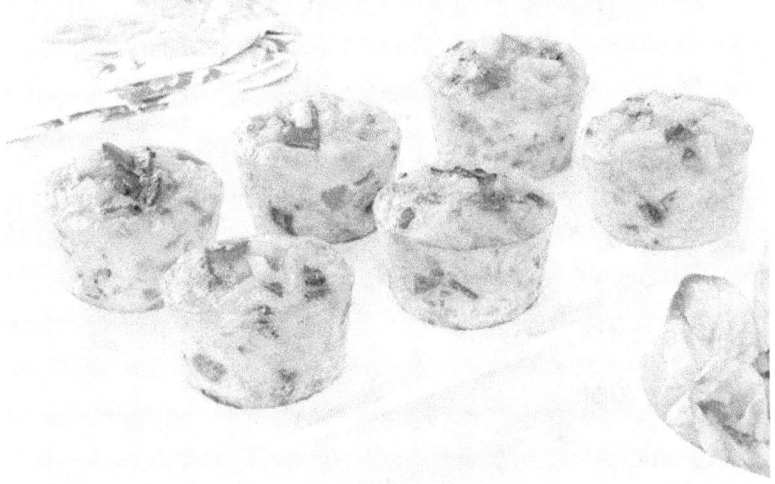

Prep Time: 15 minutes

Cooking Time: 20 minutes

Serving: 4

Ingredients:

- 8 eggs
- 8 ounce crumbled and cooked ham
- 1 cup diced red bell pepper
- 1 cup diced onion
- ¼ teaspoon salt
- 1/8 teaspoon ground black pepper
- 2 tablespoon water

Directions:

1. Pre-heat your oven to a temperature of 350 degrees Fahrenheit

2. Grease up 8 muffin cups properly
3. Take a large sized bowl and beat the eggs in your bowl
4. Add bell pepper, ham, salt, onion, black pepper and water into the egg mixture
5. Pour the mix evenly in each of the muffin tins
6. Bake them up in your pre-heated oven and for 20 minutes until the muffins are properly set
7. Serve hot!

Nutrition:

- Calories: 308
- Fat: 20.5g
- Carbohydrates: 6.8g
- Protein: 23.8g

Dinner Idea #23 - Very Romantic Mignon Fillet

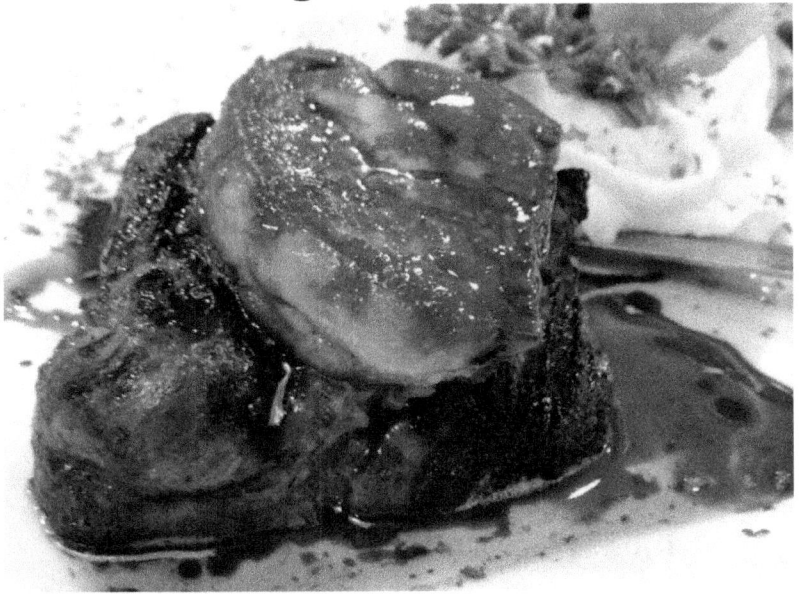

Prep Time: 5 minutes

Cooking Time: 15 minutes

Serving: 2

Ingredients:

- 8 ounce mignon steak fillets
- 2 teaspoon olive oil
- ¼ teaspoon onion powder
- Salt as needed
- Pepper as needed
- 2 tablespoon minced shallots
- 2 slices fine bacon

Directions:

1. Place a rack in the highest position inside your oven
2. Set your oven to broiling mode
3. Rub the steaks all over with your olive oil
4. Sprinkle some onion powder, pepper, and salt on top of them
5. Wrap one of the bacon slices around each of your steak and use a toothpick to secure it tightly
6. Place the prepared steaks on your broiler pan and broil for about 5-7 minutes
7. Turn them over and sprinkle some shallots
8. Broil for another 5-7 minutes
9. Once the shallots are cooked according to your preference, just serve hot!

Nutrition:

- Calories: 611
- Fat: 35g
- Carbohydrates: 2.1g
- Protein: 67g

Dinner Idea #24 - Perfectly Healthy Broccoli Soup

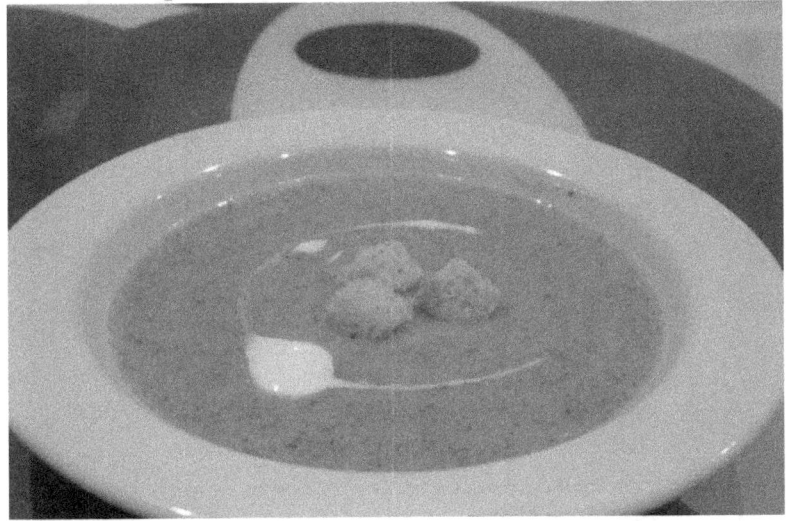

Prep Time: 15 minutes

Cooking Time: 25 minutes

Serving: 6

Ingredients:

- 1 tablespoon olive oil
- 1 chopped up large onion
- 3 peeled and chopped garlic
- 10 ounce frozen broccoli
- 1 peeled and chopped potato
- 4 cups chicken broth
- ¼ teaspoon ground nutmeg
- Salt as needed
- Pepper as needed

Directions:

1. Take a large sized saucepan and place it over medium heat
2. Heat up olive oil
3. Add garlic and onion and Sauté them until soft
4. Add in potato, broccoli, and the chicken broth
5. Bring the mix to a boil and lower down the heat
6. Simmer for about 15 minutes until the vegetables are soft
7. Take a blender and puree the mix until it has a smooth texture
8. Return the mix to your saucepan and re-heat
9. Season with some salt, nutmeg, and pepper
10. Serve hot!

Nutrition:

- Calories: 64
- Fat: 2g
- Carbohydrates: 10g
- Protein: 2.8g

Dinner Idea #25 - The Harmony Of Roast Vegetables

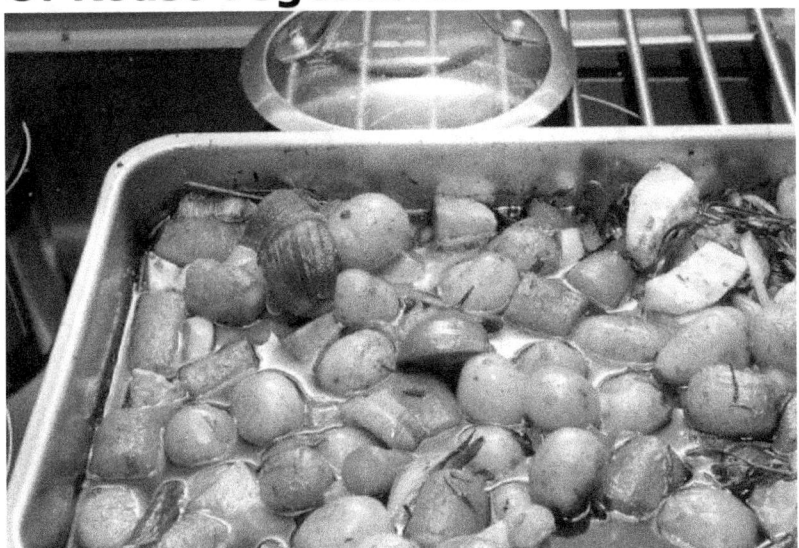

Prep Time: 25 minutes

Cooking Time: 60 minutes

Serving: 6

Ingredients:

- 2 tablespoon olive oil
- 1 large peeled yam cut up into 1-inch pieces
- 1 large parsnips peeled and cut up into 1-inch pieces
- 1 cup baby carrots
- 1 zucchini cut up into 1-inch slices
- 1 bunch fresh asparagus, trimmed up into 1-inch pieces

- ½ cup roasted red peppers cut up into 1-inch pieces
- 2 minced garlic cloves
- ¼ cup chopped up fresh basil
- ½ teaspoon kosher salt
- ½ teaspoon ground black pepper

Directions:

1. Pre-heat your oven to a temperature of 425 degrees Fahrenheit
2. Grease up 2 baking sheets with 1 tablespoon of olive oil
3. Add the parsnips, yams, and carrots onto the prepared baking sheets
4. Bake in your oven for 30 minutes
5. Add asparagus and zucchini alongside the remaining 1 tablespoon of olive oil
6. Keep baking it for 30 minutes until the vegetables are soft
7. Once soft enough, remove it from the oven and let it cool for 30 minutes your baking sheet
8. Toss the roasted peppers alongside some basil, garlic, pepper and salt in a large sized bowl
9. Combine them finely and add the roasted vegetables to the mix and toss again to mix gently
10. Serve at room temperature or chilled, depending on your preference

Nutrition:

- Calories: 191
- Fat: 5g

- Carbohydrates: 34g
- Protein: 4g

Dinner Idea #26 - Simple Currier Zucchini Soup

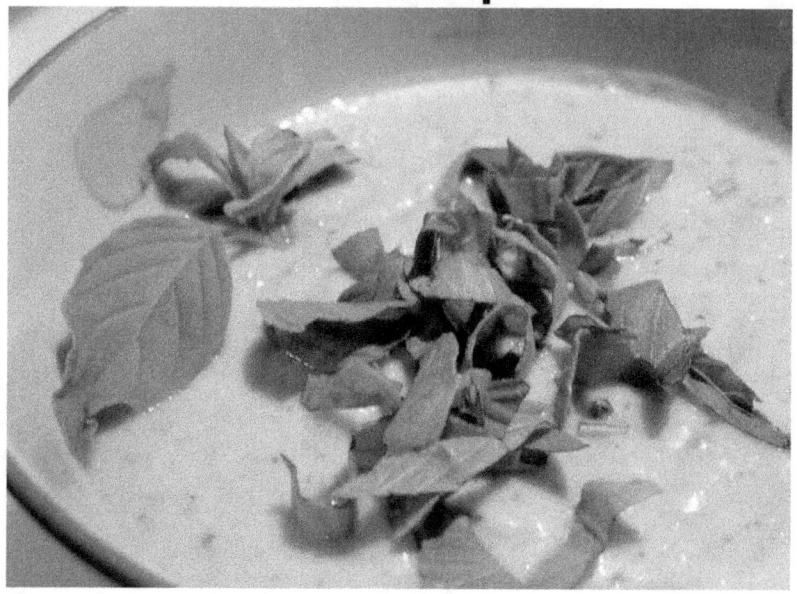

Prep Time: 25 minutes

Cooking Time: 60 minutes

Serving: 6

Ingredients:

- 2 tablespoon extra virgin olive oil
- 1 large thinly sliced halved onion
- 1 tablespoon curry powder
- Salt as needed
- 4 small sized zucchini halved up lengthwise and cut into 1-inch slices
- 1 quart chicken stock

Directions:

1. Take a large sized pot and pour in some oil
2. Stir in the onion and season the mix with salt and curry powder
3. Cook until the onion is soft
4. Stir in the zucchini and cook until soft
5. Pour in the chicken stock and bring the mix to a boil
6. Cover it up and lower down the heat
7. Simmer for 20 minutes more
8. Remove the soup from the heat and use a blender to blend the mixture until smooth
9. Serve hot!

Nutrition:

- Calories: 74
- Fat: 5.2g
- Carbohydrates: 6.3g
- Protein: 1.8g

Dinner Idea #27 - Indian Curry of Cauliflower and Potatoes

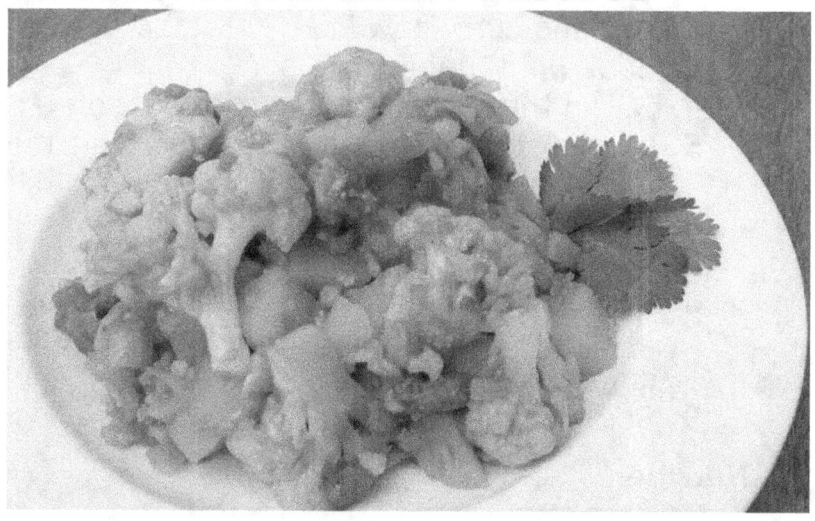

Prep Time: 15 minutes

Cooking Time: 20 minutes

Serving: 4

Ingredients:

- 1 tablespoon vegetable oil
- 1 teaspoon cumin seeds
- 1 teaspoon minced garlic
- 1 teaspoon ginger paste
- 2 medium sized cubed and peeled potatoes
- ½ teaspoon ground turmeric
- ½ teaspoon paprika
- 1 teaspoon ground cumin
- ½ teaspoon Garam masala
- Salt as needed
- 1 pound cauliflower

- 1 teaspoon chopped up fresh cilantro

Directions:

1. Take a medium sized skillet and place it over medium heat
2. Pour some oil and heat it up
3. Stir in the garlic, seeds and ginger paste
4. Cook for about 1 minute until the garlic is showing a brown texture
5. Toss in the potatoes
6. Season with some paprika, turmeric, cumin, salt and Garam masala
7. Cover it up and keep cooking for about 5-7 minutes more, making sure to stir it from time to time
8. Mix in the cilantro and cauliflower into your saucepan
9. Lower down the heat and cover it up
10. Keep stirring it from time to time and cook for another 10 minutes
11. When the cauliflower and potatoes are soft, serve hot!

Nutrition:

- Calories: 135
- Fat: 4g
- Carbohydrates: 23g
- Protein: 4g

Dinner Idea #28 - Baked Mustard Chicken With French Fried Onion

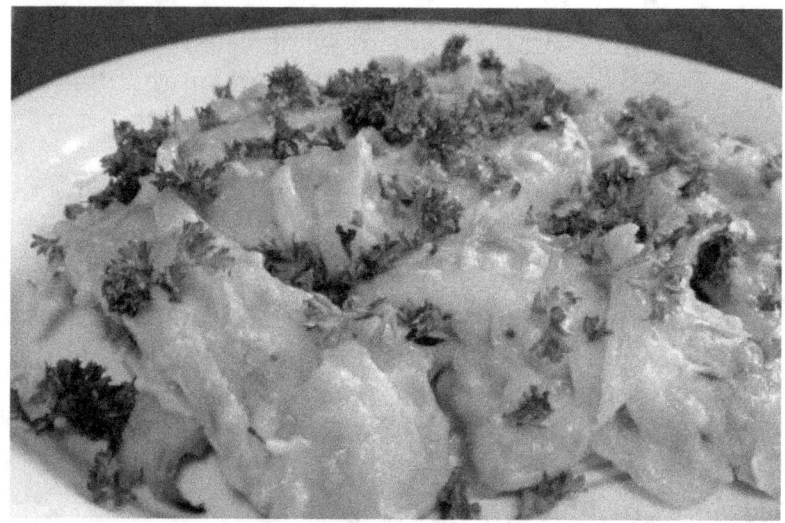

Prep Time: 15 minutes

Cooking Time: 60 minutes

Serving: 4

Ingredients:

- 4 skinless and boneless chicken breast
- 1 cup prepared mustard
- 6 ounce French-Fried onions

Directions:

1. Pre-heat your oven to a temperature of 375 degrees Fahrenheit
2. Take a shallow dish and add mustard
3. Take another shallow dish and add onions

4. Drench the chicken in mustard and make sure that it is evenly coated
5. Drench the onions in mustard then
6. Take a lightly greased 9x13 inch baking dish and place the coated chicken into the pan
7. Bake the chicken at 375 degrees Fahrenheit for about 50-60 minutes
8. Make sure that the chicken is thoroughly cooked
9. Serve

Nutrition:

- Calories: 442
- Fat: 25g
- Carbohydrates: 21g
- Protein: 30g

Dinner Idea #29 - Super Bacon Flavored Bok Choy

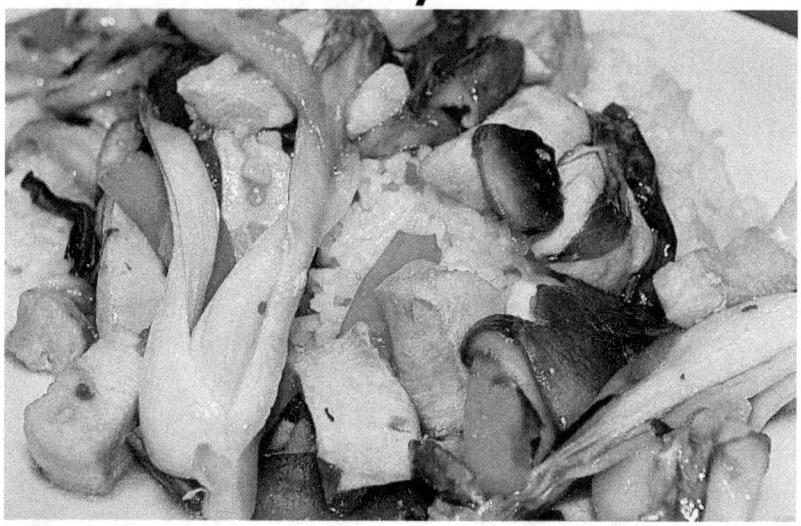

Prep Time: 15 minutes

Cooking Time: 10 minutes

Serving: 4

Ingredients:

- 4 slices chopped bacon
- 2 pounds baby bok Choy
- 1 teaspoon olive oil
- ½ small chopped red onion
- 1 teaspoon red pepper flakes
- 1 teaspoon minced garlic
- Salt as needed

Directions:

1. Take a large sized skillet and place it over medium heat

2. Fry your bacon until it is crispy
3. Remove the bacon from the pan and drain the fat
4. Keep 1 tablespoon of the grease in the skillet for future use
5. Add olive oil, red pepper flakes, onion and garlic
6. Cook and keep stirring it over medium heat until the onions are soft
7. Add bok Choy and cover it up
8. Let it cook for 5 minutes
9. Remove the lid and cook for another 2 minutes, making sure to keep stirring it until it is crunchy
10. Stir in the bacon and season it with some salt
11. Serve hot!

Nutrition:

- Calories: 97
- Fat: 5.6g
- Carbohydrates: 6.6g
- Protein: 7.1g

Dinner Idea #30 - Tasty Foiled Fish

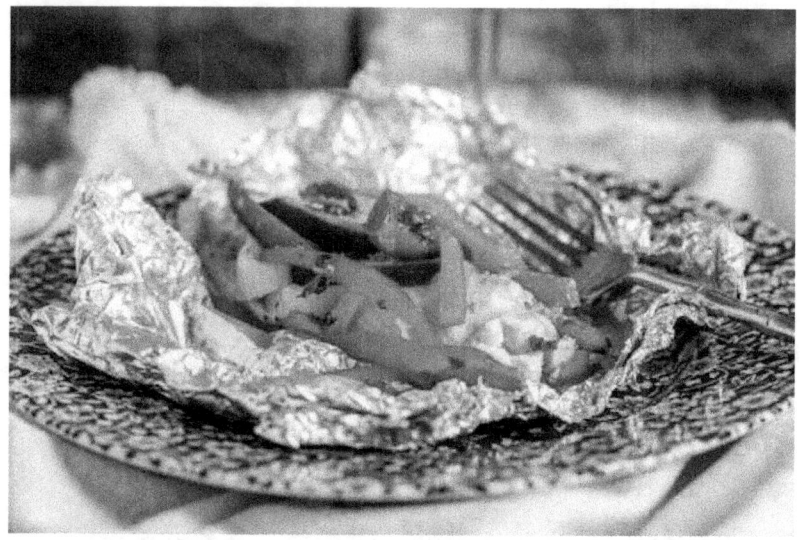

Prep Time: 10 minutes

Cooking Time: 20 minutes

Serving: 2

Ingredients:

- 2 rainbow trout fillets
- 1 tablespoon olive oil
- 2 teaspoon garlic salt
- 1 teaspoon ground black pepper
- 1 sliced fresh jalapeno pepper
- 1 sliced lemon

Directions:

1. Pre-heat your oven to a temperature of 400 degree Fahrenheit

2. Rinse your fish properly and pat it dry using a kitchen towel
3. Rub the fillets of your fish with olive oil and season them with some black pepper and garlic
4. Take a large sheet of aluminum foil and place the fillet on top of them
5. Top it up with some jalapeno slices and squeeze lemon juice from the ends of your lemon over the fish
6. Arrange the lemon slices on top of your fillets
7. Gently seal the edges of the foil to form packets
8. Place the packets on your baking sheet
9. Bake in your pre-heated oven for 20 minutes
10. The fish is done once it flakes off easily with a fork
11. Serve!

Nutrition:

- Calories: 213
- Fat: 10g
- Carbohydrates: 7.5g
- Protein: 24g

Conclusion

I would like to thank you for purchasing the book and taking the time for going through the book as well.

I do hope that this book has been helpful and you found the information contained within the scriptures useful!

Keep in mind that you are not only limited to the recipes provided in this book! Just go ahead and keep on exploring until find the perfect recipes for your next life changing 30 days!

Stay healthy and stay safe!

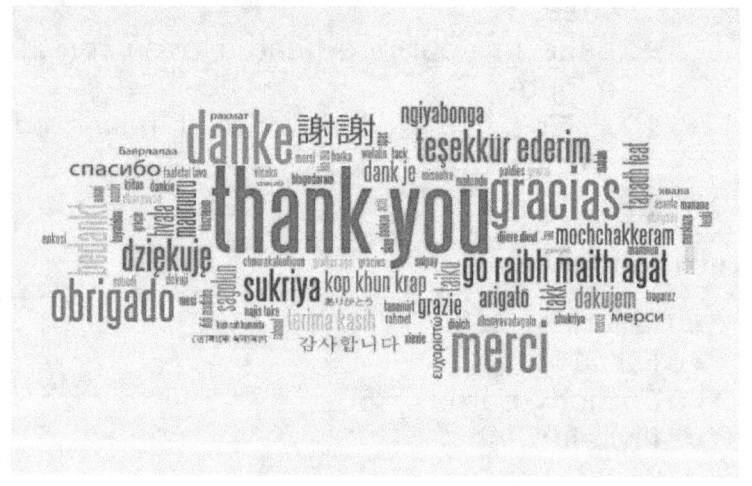

Disclaimer Notice:

Please note the information contained within this document is for educational and entertainment purposes only. Every attempt has been made to provide accurate, up to date and reliable, complete information. No warranties of any kind are expressed or implied. Readers acknowledge that the author is not engaging in the rendering of legal, financial, medical or professional advice.

By reading this document, the reader agrees that under no circumstances are we responsible for any losses, direct or indirect, which are incurred as a result of the use of information contained within this document, including, but not limited to, —errors, omissions, or inaccuracies.